Mentalization-Based Treatment for Borderline Personality Disorder

Mentalization-Based Treatment for Borderline Personality Disorder: A Practical Guide

Anthony W. Bateman, MA, FRCPsych
Consultant Psychiatrist in Psychotherapy,
Halliwick Unit, St. Ann's Hospital,
North London; and
Visiting Professor,
University College London, UK.

Peter Fonagy, PhD, FBA
Freud Memorial Professor of Psychoanalysis,
University College London; and
Chief Executive,
The Anna Freud Centre,
London, UK.

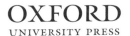

OXFORD
UNIVERSITY PRESS

OXFORD

UNIVERSITY PRESS

Great Clarendon Street, Oxford OX2 6DP

Oxford University Press is a department of the University of Oxford.
It furthers the University's objective of excellence in research, scholarship,
and education by publishing worldwide in

Oxford New York

Auckland Cape Town Dar es Salaam Hong Kong Karachi
Kuala Lumpur Madrid Melbourne Mexico City Nairobi
New Delhi Shanghai Taipei Toronto

With offices in

Argentina Austria Brazil Chile Czech Republic France Greece
Guatemala Hungary Italy Japan Poland Portugal Singapore
South Korea Switzerland Thailand Turkey Ukraine Vietnam

Oxford is a registered trade mark of Oxford University Press
in the UK and in certain other countries

Published in the United States
by Oxford University Press Inc., New York

British Library Cataloguing in Publication Data

Data available

Library of Congress Cataloging in Publication Data

Data available

Typeset by Newgen Imaging Systems (P) Ltd., Chennai, India
Printed in Great Britain
on acid-free paper by
Biddles Ltd., King's Lynn

ISBN 978–0–19–857090–5 (Pbk.)

10 9 8 7 6 5 4 3

Contents

Preface

Our first book on mentalization-based treatment (MBT), *Psychotherapy for Borderline Personality Disorder* (Bateman and Fonagy, 2004), provided an overall account of the theory and practice of our treatment for borderline patients. But it rapidly became apparent that, despite its length, depth and breadth, practitioners wanted more specificity and perhaps a little more clarity about what we actually did day by day. So we set about writing a briefer and more practical account to act as a handy companion to the original book. This is the result of our labour. We hope that this additional practical guide provides an understandable, accessible and comprehensive account of what we actually do and say in everyday clinical practice so that interested readers can move from their armchairs and seminars to their clinics and therapy sessions with confidence that what they are about to do at least resembles MBT.

But who are the interested readers we hope will gain the most? MBT is implemented within our services by nurses and other mental health professionals, few of whom are formally trained psychotherapists. This book is for them. We have tried to write it in such a way that naïve, enthusiastic practitioners, experienced in managing problematic psychiatric crises, will recognize our strategies and techniques and understand how to apply them in the treatment of borderline personality disorder. But we hope that more experienced therapists will find the account equally helpful as they contrast what they do with what we suggest they do.

Inevitably, given our own personal characteristics, what was intended to be a short pocket sized book has grown well beyond its original conception and we are grateful to Liz Allison who has patiently brought some order to our ramblings. It is her efforts that have ensured that its length is not too daunting and that it remains packed with common sense and practical information. To this end we have included many clinical examples with actual dialogue. In keeping with common practice these are often archetypal but wherever possible they include what was actually said. We have decided not to add formal references. This decision caused considerable discomfort to both of us (perhaps more so for PF!) but in the end this is a practical book, and our approach is fully referenced in our earlier book, and in many of our papers. However to help the reader with some difficult areas a few additional references are provided at the end of this book (see Further reading).

In the writing of the book we have been assisted by the continual demand for clinical seminars on MBT for which we have had to prepare presentations, workshops and practical exercises. We are grateful to all the participants who have given us their comments, suggestions, and criticisms and eventually gave us some of their experiences in actual practice. On the one hand this has helped us to clarify areas that were muddled and to elucidate our concepts in more detail, but on the other, it has exposed inconsistencies in our approach. We have tried to remedy discrepancies wherever possible but inevitably in doing so we may have created others.

We have also been assisted by senior practitioners of other therapeutic models, all of whom are exceptionally experienced in the treatment of border-line patients, who have helpfully pointed out that in our attempts to contrast mentalizing with other approaches we have fallen short in our understanding of their methods. This has led to further discussion between all of us, and it is clear that our approach shows considerable overlap with psychodynamic interpersonal therapy, cognitive analytic therapy, and transference focused therapy. Consequently practitioners trained in these models are unlikely to find our method alien. Similarly practitioners who are experienced in developing a therapeutic alliance with patients and negotiating ruptures will recognize many of our interventions. It seems that all clinicians who develop treatment plans for borderline patients are forced towards pragmatism rather than purity, and we all independently recognize the importance of focusing on therapeutic process rather than content. Specifically we would like to thank Jon Allen, Dawn Bales, John Clarkin, Glen Gabbard, John Gunderson, Sigmund Karterud, Morten Kjolbe, Otto Kernberg, Russell Meares, Anthony Ryle, Frank Yeomans, and Roel Verheul, amongst many others, for their questioning and sometimes challenging attitude about mentalizing strategies and techniques and their relationship to well-known psychotherapeutic interventions.

Finally we would like to emphasize again that our therapeutic approach lacks novelty and innovation and, to some extent, repackages commonly used therapy techniques in an attempt to harness an elemental human capacity, namely mentalizing, that is at the core of our definition of being human. We have simply made 'having a mind in mind' the object of careful study in research and in clinical practice and we hope that you will do the same as you try to understand the very painful experiences of the borderline patient. Nothing is certain in treatment of BPD and personal flexibility and ability to tolerate inconsistency are amongst the many therapist characteristics that are required for effective treatment. We ask you to bring both these traits to reading this book and to the application of our ideas and method in your clinical practice. If you do so we are sure that not only will you be able to help change minds but you will be able to delight in having your own mind changed. As we have learnt more we have modified and changed our approach, and we hope that we continue to do so, just as we hope that you will do the same as you use mentalizing as a springboard to more effective strategies.

Anthony Bateman
Peter Fonagy
London, March 2006

Foreword

I recall an incident nearly 20 years ago when I had been invited to present a workshop on borderline personality disorder in another city. My host asked if she could call the workshop, 'The Young Adult Chronic Patient'. I was a bit taken aback and replied that such a title would imply an unwarranted therapeutic nihilism. However, in retrospect, there was good reason for my host to think of such a title. From the earliest empirical research by Roy Grinker's Chicago team in the 1960s, borderline patients were found to remain pretty much the same at follow-up. They neither deteriorated nor improved.

The subsequent retrospective follow-up studies offered some hope, but the course of such patients was talked about in terms of decades rather than months or years. Moreover, analytically oriented therapists commonly struggled with such patients for 10 or 15 years, sometimes without much improvement. Because of the suicide risk in a subgroup of these patients, long-term psychoanalytically oriented hospital treatment was frequently deemed necessary as well.

Twenty years later, there has been a sea change in how we view the treatment and prognosis for borderline patients. Systematic psychotherapeutic programs have been developed, and randomized controlled trials confirm that they work. Hospitalization can largely be avoided, and results are seen in timeframes that can be measured in months and years instead of in decades. One such treatment is mentalization-based therapy (MBT), largely pioneered and developed by the authors of this first-rate new volume, Anthony Bateman and Peter Fonagy. As a follow-up to their 2004 text that laid out the theory and practice of their treatment, they now have provided us with a practical 'nuts and bolts' book for the practitioner who wishes to apply their technique in a thoughtful and systematic way.

Although the authors' approach to borderline patients has substantially altered the way that many dynamic therapists approach patients with BPD, they are remarkably modest in their claims. They stress that they are offering nothing truly novel and recognize that they are borrowing techniques that have been around a long time. They note that mentalizing is similar to the making of meaning, a cornerstone of psychodynamic therapy since its origins. However, based on their theoretical understanding of attachment and mentalizing problems intrinsic to traumatized borderline patients, they have finally honed their technique in a way that has never been so clearly expressed as in the pages of this volume.

They eschew the notion of therapeutic contracts because they know that fluctuating mentalizing capacity might well lead patients to agree to a contract in one state of mind and then subsequently find themselves in an entirely different state of mind when they chose to ignore the contract. They also advocate a kind of transparency that is unusual for dynamic therapy. They suggest writing out a formulation for the patient so that there is a genuinely collaborative effort to understand the nature of the pathology and what to do about it. Some specific components of their technique are genuinely counterintuitive for psychoanalytically trained therapists. For example, they strongly caution against making causal interventions that correlate past and present. They also advocate the postponement of transference work rather than interpreting what appears to be the self-object dyad enacted in the therapeutic relationship. They emphasize that the therapist should stay with conscious content rather than exploring unconscious concerns, and they prefer process to content as the discourse between therapist and patient. Interventions should be brief and to the point. One avoids activating the attachment system in one's comments. The focus must be on affect in the current context. One avoids a judgemental attitude about self-harm and suicide by focusing on what is going on in the patient's mind instead of confronting behaviour. Experienced therapists will have to be willing to give up some sacred cows. For example, the goal is not to provide insight!

In this latest contribution, Bateman and Fonagy provide a good deal of help for the floundering therapist who struggles to sort out the chaos of borderline psychopathology. Therapists must do their best to construct and reconstruct an image of the patient in the therapist's mind. Therapists must also understand themselves and must approach the therapy with a measure of humility. A 'not knowing' stance is essential. Patient and therapist share their respective points of view without asserting who is right and who is wrong. Therapists need to be wary of their own tendency to fall into an anti-mentalizing position. They monitor their countertransference for signs of enactments, and are willing to 'stop, rewind, and explore' when necessary. Much as Kohut recommended in the early 1970s, Bateman and Fonagy suggest that therapists should freely acknowledge their own role in any ruptures in the therapeutic relationship. Patient and therapist carefully review what happened prior to the rupture and then do their best to repair the damage.

There is a splendid chapter on assessing mentalization. The process is no easy matter, as mentalization is context dependent and may appear to be dramatically different from session to session when treating borderline patients. Nevertheless, a detailed list of questions will guide the therapist in the direction of making a reasonable assessment of the patient's overall capacity for imagining there own mind and that of others. The authors also include an array of figures and tables to make the book more reader friendly.

I particularly liked the final chapter on frequently asked questions because by the time I got to the end of the book, a number of these questions were haunting me. What is the overlap between supportive therapy and MBT? Is MBT mother-blaming? Is mentalizing a common factor in all therapies? Many more questions are thoughtfully addressed by the authors, who have impressively mentalized their readers' internal state as they near the end of the book.

We all learned the hard way that one cannot learn psychotherapy from a book alone. Nevertheless, 'how-to' books like this one provide the foundation on which we build knowledge learned from supervisors and from our most helpful teachers, our patients. This book will serve both beginning and experienced therapists well in offering an inspired road map on the challenging journey we take with borderline patients. I commend the authors for their cartography skills and their wisdom.

Glen O. Gabbard, M.D.
Brown Foundation Chair of Psychoanalysis
and Professor of Psychiatry
Baylor College of Medicine
July 2006

Chapter 1

Introduction to mentalization

This chapter will define the concept of mentalization and will link it to concepts such as empathy and psychological mindedness that may be more familiar to clinicians. After defining the concept we will explore a range of clinical applications and link the concept to the nature of psychological therapy.

What is mentalizing?

Mentalizing simply implies a focus on mental states in oneself or in others, particularly in explanations of behaviour. That mental states influence behaviour is beyond question. Beliefs, wishes, feelings and thoughts, whether inside or outside our awareness, determine what we do.

Explanations of behaviour in terms of others' mental states are relatively vulnerable compared with explanations that refer to aspects of the physical environment. The latter are far less ambiguous because the physical world is less readily changeable. When taking a mentalizing stance the mere contemplation of alternative possibilities may lead to a change in beliefs. A focus on mind leads to far more uncertain conclusions than a focus on physical circumstances, because it concerns a mere representation of reality rather than reality itself. We may act according to wrong beliefs about others' mental states in a particular situation, sometimes with tragic consequences. In the middle ages if people believed that a person was possessed by the devil it was sufficient grounds for burning them alive; nowadays if a person believes that someone is a terrorist it may also at times be sufficient grounds for taking that person's life.

Mentalization is a mostly preconscious, imaginative mental activity. It is imaginative because we have to imagine what other people might be thinking or feeling. It lacks homogeneity because each person's history and capacity to imagine may lead them to different conclusions about the mental states of others. We may sometimes need to make the same kind of imaginative leap to understand our own experiences, particularly in relation to emotionally charged issues or irrational, nonconsciously driven reactions.

To adopt a mentalizing stance, to conceive of oneself and others as having a mind, requires a representational system for mental states. Although mentalizing probably involves numerous cortical systems, it is certainly associated with activation in the middle prefrontal areas of the brain, probably the paracingulate area (Gallagher and Frith, 2003). It is likely that several brain systems are involved in different aspects of mentalizing, including those underpinning attentional processes and emotional reactions (see Fonagy and Bateman, in press).

A focus on mental states seems self-evident for those involved in treating individuals with mental disorder. Yet even those of us engaged in daily clinical work can all too easily forget that our clients have minds. For example, many biological psychiatrists are happier to think in terms of neurotransmitter imbalance than distorted expectations or self-representation. Parents with children who have psychological problems often prefer to understand these either in terms of genetic predispositions or direct consequences of the child's social environment. Even psychotherapists can make unwarranted assumptions about what their patients' theory about their illness and its treatment might be and their interventions indicate that they might have lost touch with the actual subjective experience of their patient. As Dennett (1987) aptly put it, 'How could anything be more familiar, and at the same time more weird, than a mind?'

Allen (in press) suggests that we should favour the word 'mentalizing' over 'mentalization' to indicate that this is something we either do or fail to do.

Box 1.1 **What is mentalizing?**

- Mentalizing may be defined as perceiving and interpreting behaviour as conjoined with intentional mental states
- Mentalizing is based on assumptions that mental states influence human behaviour
- Mentalizing requires a careful analysis of the circumstances of actions
- Mentalizing requires a careful analysis of prior patterns of behaviour
- Mentalizing requires an analysis of the experiences the individual has been exposed to
- Mentalizing, while it demands complex cognitive processes, is mostly preconscious
- Mental states (e.g. beliefs), unlike most aspects of the physical world, are readily changeable
- A focus on the products of mentalizing is a more error-prone process than the focus on physical circumstance because it concerns a mere representation of reality rather than reality itself
- Mentalizing is an imaginative mental activity

Allen defines mentalizing as 'perceiving and interpreting behaviour as conjoined with intentional mental states'. It is a profoundly social construct in the sense that we are attentive to the mental states of those we are with, physically or psychologically. Equally we can temporarily lose awareness of them as 'minds' and even momentarily treat them as physical objects. Elsewhere we have speculated that for physical violence to be possible, we have to deliberately foreclose the possibility that the individual we violate has a mind (Fonagy, 2004), either by considering the person as a physical object or as a member of a large alien social group but not as an individual with specific concerns and beliefs.

Mentalizing and emotional life

Psychoanalytic colleagues have criticized our emphasis on mentalization for being overly focused on cognition. This is a misapprehension. Mentalization is procedural, mostly non-conscious. That is to say, it occurs pretty much out of our conscious control, automatically, in response to the innumerable social events that occur around us. It is not merely cognitive and certainly the cognitive aspects are closely tied to the affective ones. Mentalizing is for the most part an intuitive rapid emotional reaction. Feelings within ourselves and our impressions of others' feelings provide us with considerable information about the mental states that underpin behaviour (Damasio, 2003). Probably our experience of the affective tone of an interaction can lead us to relatively complex choices between sets of beliefs. For example, if we experience an individual as threatening this may lead us to formulate relatively complex theories about their hostile intentions.

Mentalizing also helps us to regulate our emotions. Emotions relate directly to our achievement of, or failure to achieve, specific wishes or desires. Thus, beliefs about having achieved goals or desires will inevitably generate an emotional response. Children can understand emotional states before they can understand knowledge or beliefs. Infants are predisposed to learn about the world from a trusted adult (Gergely and Csibra, 2003). The emotional tone of the adult in relation to a specific experience can offer the infant a clue about whether it is safe, and more generally the child expects to receive all types of knowledge about the world through the mind of a trusted other.

It is easy to overlook the non-conscious aspect of mentalizing. For something as simple as maintaining a dialogue we need to monitor our conversational partner's state of mind. Perceiving and responding fluidly to their emotions ensures that our conversation goes smoothly. In an ingenious investigation, Steimer-Krause and colleagues (1990) demonstrated that we automatically mirror our interlocutors' emotional states, adjusting our posture, facial expressions and tone of voice in the process. Thus it is possible to diagnose the characteristic flattened affect of chronic schizophrenia from the facial expressions of a non-schizophrenic person engaged in an ordinary conversation with an individual who has a diagnosis of schizophrenia, even though the non-schizophrenic person is unaware of this diagnosis.

The implicit mentalization of one's own actions is an emotional state (Damasio, 2003) characterized by a sense of oneself as an agent (Marcel, 2003). In general, awareness of our behaviour as driven by mental states gives us the sense of continuity and control that generates the subjective experience of agency or 'I-ness' which is at the very core of a sense of identity. We have described the simultaneous experience and knowledge of emotion as mentalized affectivity. Many dynamic therapies aim to enable consciousness of one's affects whilst remaining in that emotional state and understanding that state as meaningful. We believe that mentalized affectivity is crucial to the regulation of emotion, that is, without it the capacity to identify, modulate and express one's affects is definitely curtailed (Fonagy *et al.*, 2002). Allen (2006) concludes that mentalizing implicitly entails a prereflective sense of connectedness to the agentive self: 'one has a sense of oneself as an emotional, engaged agent'.

Related concepts

Empathy

Many, particularly those with a self-psychology or client-centred therapy background, think that empathy overlaps or is even synonymous with the concept of mentalizing. The strict definition of the concept of empathy is 'identification with and understanding of another's feelings and motives or the attribution of one's own feelings to an object' (American Heritage Dictionary). But the term is most commonly used in a narrow sense indicating awareness of and resonance with an emotional state of distress in another.

Gallese and colleagues (2004) built a strong case suggesting that empathy is mediated by a specific neural mirror mechanism that allows us to directly understand the meaning of others' actions and emotions by internally replicating these. They suggest that for both actions and emotions, specific neural systems exist where the same neurones are activated both when a person performs a particular action and when s/he observes another individual performing a similar action. The implication of this discovery according to Gallese and colleagues is that we have a direct experiential grasp of the mind of others and do not have to infer their self-states through conceptual reasoning.

The original evidence for this supposition came from macaque monkeys, but more recent studies have found evidence from human mirror neurone systems that 'resonate' in response to a wide range of actions. The data suggest that when we watch someone perform an action this activates part of the same motor circuits that are recruited when we ourselves perform that action. Similarly, certain brain regions (the insula) that are activated during the experience of specific emotions (disgust) are also activated during the observation of someone else's facial expression of the same emotion (Wicker et al., 2003). This suggests that understanding basic aspects of social cognition depends on activation of neural structures normally involved in our own personally experienced actions and emotions.

This formulation of empathy is too mechanistic and speaks to slightly different phenomena than the mentalization concept. However, Preston and de Waal (2002) advanced a theory of empathy based on findings concerning mirror neurones, all of which involve matching the state of subject and object. Cognitive empathy as defined by these workers goes beyond emotional matching and requires an imaginative capacity working with representations of shared experience. While mentalization appears to us to be an independent brain system from the mirror neuron system, the higher order forms of empathy described by Preston and de Waal clearly overlap with the concept as advanced in this volume.

On balance we consider that the term empathy, as commonly used, has two fundamental limitations that preclude us from simply adopting the term. First, the concept of empathy or simulation as used by Gallese and colleagues assumes an awareness of a self-state that can be mapped on to the state of the other in order to apprehend their state, that is, mentalization of the self must be seen as a precursor. Second, empathy, as Gallese and colleagues consider it, specifically precludes a reflective or conceptual phase and emphasizes an immediate preconceptual awareness of correspondence.

Psychological mindedness

Appelbaum (1973) defines psychological mindedness as a capacity to relate actions to thoughts and feelings. This definition is very similar to Dennett's definition of the intentional stance as interpreting people's actions in terms of mental states. However, the psychotherapy researchers McCallum and Piper (1996) have used the term to refer to the specific ability to identify dynamic or intrapsychic components and to relate them to a person's difficulties.

With notable exceptions (e.g. Farber, 1985) psychological mindedness is a construct restricted to the capacity to mentalize the self. Thus whilst empathy principally concerns awareness of others in mental state terms, psychological mindedness, probably because of its roots in psychological therapy, is used generally as a mentalizing approach to self-understanding.

It is not surprising that there is a close link between the notion of receptivity to insight included in the concept of mentalizing and the concept of psychological mindedness. It is possible that this association is simply an artefact of the origin of both constructs within the psychoanalytic approach. Some philosophers of mind have suggested that Freud's concept of psychic determinism is tantamount to extending the notion of mentalization to a non-conscious part of the mind, that is, unconscious beliefs are as powerful determinants of action as conscious ones (Hopkins, 1992; Wollheim, 1995). In any event, psychological mindedness is the facet of mentalizing that indicates a predisposition to explanation of behaviour in terms of determinants that are external to the subject's awareness.

Mind-mindedness

The attachment field rapidly adopted mentalization as a construct. Two findings linked security of attachment to mentalization. First, a relatively high manifest ability for mentalization on the part of the parent in relation to their own attachment history was found to predict security of attachment in the child (Fonagy et al., 1991; Slade et al., 2005). Second, children with secure attachment histories acquire mentalization earlier (Fonagy et al., 1997; Meins et al., 2002).

A number of laboratories have produced findings linking mentalization to attachment (David Oppenheim in Haifa, Elizabeth Meins in Durham, England and Arietta Slade in New York). Elizabeth Meins coined the term 'maternal mind-mindedness' to denote her observation that mothers who used more mental state language in their 'conversations' with their six-month-old infants were more likely to have infants securely attached to them at one year (Meins et al., 2002). Similarly, Oppenheim (Koren-Karie et al., 2002) found more mental state language in mothers' narration of a video recording of their interaction with their child when the child was securely attached.

These findings point to mind-mindedness as an important facilitator of the creation of secure attachment bonds. Obviously maternal mind-mindedness is mentalization of the child in a very specific context of the attachment relationship. Having been felt to be the object of someone's mentalizing obviously enhances mentalizing capacities in the young child.

Mindfulness

Mindfulness is a construct originating in Zen Buddhist philosophy. It implies an acute orientation to current experience. Zen teaches that each moment is complete and perfect by itself and acceptance, toleration and validation rather than change should be the therapeutic focus (Hayes *et al.*, 2004). In its original sense it is not specific to mental states but as Allen (in press) points out, some facets of mindfulness imply sensitivity to psychological processes. The central construct is the recognition that thoughts are just thoughts and that they are not 'you' or 'reality'. This recognition can free the patient from the distorted reality that thoughts can create.

Mindfulness has found an important area of application in cognitive-behavioural approaches that include dialectical behaviour therapy (DBT, Linehan, 1987) and a form of cognitive-behavioural therapy for depression aiming to reduce the likelihood of recurrence (Teasdale *et al.*, 2000). Thus mindfulness is related to but is also a broader concept than mentalization. It reflects an attitude of openness which is indeed also implied by the mentaliza-tion construct. It is, however, equally applicable as currently construed to the physical as to the mental world.

Symbolization, transitional space and the 'third position'

Mentalizing as a construct is very close to meaning-making. In fact, when cli-nicians talk about symbolization they mostly mean not the capacity to use one object to represent another (the strict sense of the term) but rather a fluency in mental state language. Thus the absence of symbolic capacity, concreteness, is mostly used to describe narratives that lack reference to internal states in accounts of behaviour and privilege physical circumstances. Symbolization overlaps with what we have referred to as the capacity to play with reality; that is, treat reality as a representation.

Symbolization, thus defined, combines two modes of functioning that ante-date it developmentally. These modes are often offered in psychoanalytic texts as indications of the failure of symbolization (see Box 1.2). The psychic equi-valence mode common in two-to-three year old children collapses the differ-entiation between inner and outer, symbol and symbolized, and internal and external reality. Psychic equivalence dominates the concrete understanding of mental states discussed in detail in Chapter 5. The alternative, the pretend mode, assumes no connection between internal and external reality and any forced contact between the two inhibits imagination. Pretend mode thinking links may underpin much of what we later describe as pseudo-mentalizaton where mental states are described which have little or no connection with actual reality.

In mentalization these two modes of representation are integrated so that subjectivity closely represents but also remains decoupled from physical real-ity. A similar in-between state is implied by Winnicott's notion of transitional

---

Box 1.2 The modes of subjective experience that antedate mentalization

◆ Psychic equivalence:
  • Mind-world isomorphism; mental reality = outer reality → internal has status and power of the external
  • When frightening thoughts are felt as real the subjective experience of mind can be terrifying (flashbacks)
  • Intolerance of alternative perspectives ('if I think you had your door shut because you want to reject me, then you want to reject me')
  • Self-related negative cognitions may be felt to be *too real*

◆ Pretend mode:
  • Ideas form no bridge between inner and outer reality; mental world decoupled from external reality
  • Linked with emptiness, meaninglessness and dissociation in the wake of trauma
  • Endless inconsequential talk of thoughts and feelings in therapy
  • Marked by simultaneously held contradictory beliefs
  • Frequently affects do not match the content of thoughts

---

space (Winnicott, 1971). Ogden's (1985) writing on potential space describes a very similar construct. All these notions imply the ability to move away from physical reality sufficiently to be able to manipulate it but not so far away that the correspondence between the real world and the mental representation is lost. There is a playfulness and humour implied in these constructs, an attitude that is implicit in many aspects of mentalization but certainly goes way beyond. Humour and playfulness are necessary in our view to enhancing mentalization, partly to demonstrate that mental states are inherently modifiable and malleable. This approach to subjectivity produces a creative stance towards the world.

Clinical implications of the focus on mentalization

Given the generality of our definition of mentalization, most mental disorders will inevitably involve some difficulties with mentalization. In fact we can conceive of most mental disorder as the mind misinterpreting its own experience of itself, thus ultimately a disorder of mentalization.

An aspect of treatment-resistant chronic depression is very low self-esteem driven by an apparent bias in the direction of negative self-appraisal. One way to think about this bias may be in terms of the status our mind assigns to fleeting negative thoughts. Recognizing these as 'only ideas' might help protect us from their implications. However, the same fleeting negative self-evaluations in the mode of psychic equivalence are experienced with the full force of physical reality. Thus, chronically depressed individuals may not have representations of themselves that are more negative than that of anyone else; rather, they experience ordinary negative self-evaluations (which we all have) in a psychic equivalent mode and they feel these thoughts with the full force of reality. Distortions in mentalizing may account for other kinds of psychological disturbance. For example, anxiety could be seen as assessing risk or danger to self in a psychic equivalent mode.

There are two key issues here. The first key issue is that when we talk about failures of mentalization we are inevitably discussing a dual problem. First, and often less noticeable, is the dysfunction of mentalization, a loss of some aspect of the capacity to see the other fully as a person or subjectivity as amenable to re-presentation. The second part of the dual problem is a complication of the first, the re-emergence of non-mentalizing modes of thinking, variously referred to as concreteness, impulsivity, affect dysregulation and propensity for acting out, etc. These, often correlated, mental phenomena not only point to the absence of a regulatory function but also a dysregulated state caused by non-mentalizing modes of subjectivity. Thus if internal experiences are felt to be too real (as in flashbacks) their emotional impact will inevitably be far greater. The loss of mentalizing function manifests itself as the re-emergence of developmentally earlier mental structures that come to replace the non-functioning systems and the problems these create within an already vulnerable mental world. A person who is unable to mentalize will be far more vulnerable and disequilibrated by apparently slight changes in conditions.

The second key issue is that notwithstanding that mental disorder when looked at from a psychological perspective will always entail a disorder of mentalization, not all mental disorders are usefully looked at in this way. The issue here is not whether a disorder can be redescribed in terms of the functioning of mentalization but rather whether the dysfunction of mentalization is core to the disorder and a focus on mentalization is heuristically valid; that is, provides an appropriate domain for therapeutic intervention. For example, in the case of autism, patients have been shown to suffer more or less complete mind-blindness (Baron-Cohen *et al.*, 2000). Whether this provides an appropriate focus for interventions is currently an open question.

We believe that trauma victims often experience partial failures of mentalization. As Allen (2000) has demonstrated, in this case a focus on mentalization can provide an extremely useful background. What has been described as desensitization to memories of trauma may, for example, be equally well or better considered as helping to turn unmentalized images into mentalized traumatic memories.

In disorders that involve misrepresentation of mental contents, as for example in typical misattributions associated with conduct problems (Lochman and Dodge, 1994), in many cases therapeutic approaches may address specific attributions rather than the generic capacity to mentalize.

In the case of borderline personality disorder as we will describe in the next chapter, mentalization may be suppressed by a combination of trauma history and the related hyperactivation of the attachment system, as well as a background high-level arousal. A focus on the capacity to mentalize in the face of the challenges created by a therapeutic relationship may provide a sensible entry point for treatment of BPD. Children who are emotionally abused (exposed to harmful parenting) are by definition in a family environment that inadequately mentalizes them. Again in such cases an approach aimed at generally enhancing mentalization can be seen as providing a good basis for therapy.

Conclusions

Mentalizing is the key social-cognitive capacity that has allowed human beings to create effective social groups. Mentalization is acquired in a social context although the predisposition for it must be inherited, just like the propensity for language. As a psychological scientific construct mentalization is not new and several related constructs help in completing a description of the range of phenomena that the application of the concept in a psychotherapeutic context will entail. Our approach assumes that dysfunctions of mentalization not only create major relationship problems but also lead to subjective distress which can result in self-harm and suicidality. The close interface between attachment processes and mentalizing is the key to this. Disturbed relationships both undermine and are undermined by failures of mentalization. We therefore argue that the correction of some of these relational malfunctions can be achieved by assisting patients in the recovery of mentalizing.

Chapter 2

Using the mentalization model to understand severe personality disorder

Overview of the developmental model

Vulnerability factors

Our theoretical understanding of borderline personality disorder is rooted in John Bowlby's attachment theory (1988) and its elaboration by developmental psychologists (Main, Sroufe, Tronick, Lyons-Ruth), especially George Gergely and John Watson's work with contingency theory (Gergely and Watson, 1999; Watson, 2001). According to attachment theory the development of the self occurs in the affect regulatory context of early relationships. Not surprisingly then, disorganization of the attachment system results in disorganization of self-structure.

We assume that to achieve normal self-experience the infant requires his emotional signals to be accurately or contingently mirrored by an attachment figure. The mirroring must be 'marked' (e.g. exaggerated); in other words slightly distorted, if the infant is to understand the caregiver's display as part of his emotional experience rather than an expression of hers. This may be a behavioural analogue to the containment concept. We have collected evidence to suggest that the absence of marked contingent mirroring is associated with the later development of disorganized attachment. Infants whose attachment has been observed to be disorganized exhibit behaviours like freezing (dissociation) and self harm and go on to develop oppositional highly controlling behavioural tendencies in middle childhood.

We assume, as suggested by Winnicott (1956), that when a child cannot develop a representation of his own experience through mirroring (the self), he internalizes the image of the caregiver as part of his self-representation. We have called this discontinuity within the self the alien self. We understand the controlling behaviour of children with a history of disorganized attachment as persistence of a pattern analogous to projective identification where the experience of incoherence within the self is reduced through externalization.

The intense need for the caregiver characteristic of separation anxiety in middle childhood that is associated with disorganized attachment reflects the need for the caregiver as a vehicle for externalization of the alien part of the self rather than simply an insecure attachment relationship.

The experience of fragmentation within the self-structure is reduced by the concurrent development of 'mentalization', the capacity to represent interpersonal experience as well as self-experience in mental state terms. Understanding the behaviour of others in terms of their likely thoughts, feelings, wishes and desires is a major developmental achievement which biologically originates in the context of the attachment relationship. One's understanding of others critically depends on one's own mental states being adequately understood by caring, non-threatening adults. This is best achieved through a secure, playful child–caregiver relationship that invites playfulness in relations to feelings and thoughts, beliefs and desires and enhances the firm establishment of mentalizing.

Activating factors

Several factors can disrupt the normal deployment of mentalizing. Most important amongst these is psychological trauma early or late in childhood. We have found extensive evidence to suggest that childhood attachment trauma undermines the capacity to think about mental states in giving narrative accounts of one's past attachment relationships and even in trying to identify the mental states associated with specific facial expressions. This may be due to; (a) the defensive inhibition of the capacity to think about others' thoughts and feelings in the face of the experience of genuine malevolent intent of others and the overwhelming vulnerability of the child; (b) early excessive stress may distort the functioning of arousal mechanisms inhibiting orbito-frontal cortical activity (mentalizing) at far lower levels of risk than would be normally the case; and (c) any trauma arouses the attachment system (seeking for protection) and attachment trauma may do so chronically. In seeking proximity to the traumatizing attachment figure as a consequence of trauma, the child may naturally be further traumatized. The prolonged activation of the attachment system may be an additional problem as the arousal of attachment may have specific inhibitory consequences for mentalization in addition to that which might be expected as a consequence of increased emotional arousal (see Chapter 3). Further, the child in 'identifying with the aggressor' as a way of gaining illusory control over the abuser may internalize the intent of the aggressor into the alien (dissociated) part of the self. While this might offer temporary relief, the destructive intent of the abuser will in this way come to be experienced from within rather than outside of the self and an unbearable experience of self-hatred might be the consequence.

Phenomenology

The phenomenology of BPD is the consequence of: (a) the attachment-related inhibition of mentalization; (b) the re-emergence of modes of experiencing internal reality that ante-date the developmental emergence of mentalization; and (c) the constant pressure for projective identification, the re-externalization of the self-destructive alien self. Taking these in turn, individuals with border-line personality disorder are 'normal' mentalizers except in the context of attachment relationships. They tend to misread minds, both their own and those of others, when emotionally aroused and as their relationship with another moves into the sphere of attachment the intensification of relation-ships means that their ability to think about the mental state of another can rapidly disappear. When this happens, prementalistic modes of organizing subjectivity emerge, which have the power to disorganize these relationships and destroy the coherence of self-experience that the narrative provided by normal mentalization generates.

In this way mentalization gives way to psychic equivalence, which clinicians normally consider under the heading of concreteness of thought. No altern-ative perspectives are possible. There is a suspension of the experience of 'as if' and everything appears to be 'for real'. This can add drama as well as risk to interpersonal experience and the exaggerated reaction of patients is justified by the seriousness with which they suddenly experience their own and others' thoughts and feelings.

Conversely, thoughts and feelings can come to be almost dissociated to the point of near meaninglessness. In these states patients can discuss experiences without contextualizing these in any kind of physical or material reality. Attempting psychotherapy with patients who are in this mode can lead the therapist to lengthy but inconsequential discussions of internal experience that has no link to genuine experience.

Finally, early modes of conceptualizing action in terms of that which is apparent can come to dominate motivation. Within this mode there is a primacy of the physical, and experience is only felt to be valid when its consequences are apparent to all. Affection, for example, is only true when accompanied by physical expression. The most disruptive feature of border-line cognition is the apparently unstoppable tendency to create unacceptable experience within the other. The externalization of the alien self is desirable for the child with a disorganized attachment but is a matter of life and death for the traumatized individual who has internalized the abuser as part of the self. The alternative to projective identification is the destruction of the self in a teleological mode, that is, physically, by self-harm and suicide. These and other actions can also serve to create a terrified alien self in the other—therapist, friend, parent—who becomes the vehicle for what is emotionally unbearable. The need for this other can become overwhelming and an adhesive, addictive pseudo-attachment to this individual may develop.

Disorganization of attachment

In the last chapter we touched on evidence suggesting that the parent's capacity for mentalization is associated with secure attachment in the child. The converse of this is that low levels of mentalization generate insecure and perhaps disorganized attachment. For example, in a study recently reported by Arietta Slade and colleagues, low levels of mentalization of her child by the mother were associated with maternal behaviours known and shown in the study to generate an increased likelihood of disorganized attachment in the infant characterized by paradoxical response to the attachment figure (e.g. hiding from attachment figure on reunion) (Slade *et al.*, 2005). Disorganized attachment in infancy is very likely to be associated with self-harming behaviours, propensity for dissociation, aggressive and potentially violent behaviour (Lyons-Ruth, 1996; Sroufe, 2005). Although the underlying mechanisms are not yet known, we have suggested that poor mentalization of the infant by the mother undermines the healthy development of some of the infant's social cognitive capacities, particularly the regulation of affect and the efficient functioning of focused attention (Fonagy and Target, 2002). Poor affect regulation and attentional control undermine parent–infant interaction, which in turn can undermine attachment processes, leading to further disorganization of the attachment relationship.

Box 2.1 **Working with disorganized attachment**

Practice points

- With individuals whose attachment relationships have been disorganized we may anticipate quite severe problems in affect regulation and attentional control along with profound dysfunctions of attachment relationships
- Exploratory psychotherapy techniques are likely to dysregulate the patient's affect
- It is wise to anticipate difficulties in effortful control (the inhibition of prepotent responses)

Disorganized attachment and the disorganization of the self: the alien self

If the social processes that normally enable a person to develop a sense of himself as an agent fail, there are important complications for that person's development. Infants are constitutionally primed to expect to find a version of their internal states mirrored by their caregivers. These mirroring responses are necessary to help them learn to represent their internal states both to themselves and others (Fonagy *et al.*, 2002; Gergely and Watson, 1996). If a small child does not have access to an adult who is able to recognize and respond to his internal states he will find it very difficult to make his own experience meaningful. Ideally the child needs an adult to reflect his state of mind in a manner that indicates to the child that it is not the caregiver's but the child's mental state that is being expressed. We think of this as 'marked mirroring' and consider it analogous to what a good psychotherapist does in reflecting the patient's affect—combining accuracy of mirroring with a sense that she is coping with the patient's experience.

If the adult's mirroring reactions do not reflect the infant's experience accurately, the infant is nevertheless forced to use these incongruent reflections to assist in organizing internal states. Unfortunately, as they do not map sufficiently well on to the child's experience, the self will be prone to disorganization, that is, incoherence and fragmentation. This phenomenon was first noted by Winnicott (1967) and is also implied in Kohut's (1971) concept of an enfeebled self. Both these psychoanalysts noted that incongruent mirroring forces the child to internalize representations of the parent's state rather than a usable version of his own experience. We have suggested that this creates an alien experience within the self (Fonagy *et al.*, 1995). The subjective experience that corresponds to this may be a sense of having feelings and ideas that are 'known as one's own' but do not 'feel like one's own'.

As partial failure of maternal mentalization of the infant is probably ubiquitous, it is likely that all of us have such non-integrated parts of the self to a degree. It seems that states of mind that are not felt to fit coherently into a self-structure are nevertheless integrated into it by the capacity for mentalization. We smooth over the discontinuities by creating an intentional narrative (imagining that we always intended to do whatever it was because we had felt/thought/wished for, etc.). In children whose attachment history is one of disorganization because of the hostile, frightening or fearful behaviour of their caregiver, the part of the self-representation that is poorly linked to the self-structure is expected to be more extensive. Further, because the capacities required for mentalization are compromised, the discontinuities of the self will be more evident more of the time. Without mentalization it is difficult to create an illusion of coherence through the attribution of agency.

Controlling internal working model

The sense of agency that we experience by attributing mental states normally lends coherence and psychological meaning to our actions, our sense of self and ultimately to our life. Individuals whose capacity for mentalization is not well developed may be forced to use controlling and manipulative strategies to restore the coherence of the self.

We assume that incongruent or alien aspects of the self are experienced as belonging to the attachment figure in order to create an illusion of coherence. Attachment research has demonstrated that disorganized attachment in infancy is often followed by extremely controlling and dominating behaviour in middle childhood (Solomon and George, 1999). In the clinical literature the process is often described as 'evocatory projective identification' (Spillius, 1992). The attachment figure is manipulated into feeling the emotions that have been internalized as part of the self but are not entirely felt to be of the self.

It is helpful to remember that this type of self-protective manoeuvre is not about shedding feelings that the individual cannot acknowledge. It is about protecting the self from the experience of incongruence or incoherence that has the potential to generate far greater anxiety. From a clinical perspective, therefore, drawing the patient's attention to this process will rarely have the desired consequence of bringing it to an end. For example, if a person persistently behaves in a frustrating way in order to create anger and resentment in the person they are with, this behaviour is not driven by the wish not to acknowledge anger against the object. Rather, it is the experience of anger within and against the self that creates the unbearable state of mind which is dealt with through projective identification.

Box 2.2 Discontinuity in the self

Practice points

- The therapist should be alert to subjective experiences indicating discontinuities in self structure (e.g. a sense of having a wish/belief/feeling which does not 'feel like their own')
- It is inappropriate to see these states of minds as if they were manifestations of a dynamic unconscious and as indications of the 'true' but 'disguised' or 'repressed' wish/belief/feeling of the patient
- The discontinuity in the self will have an aversive aspect to most patients leading to a sense of discontinuity in identity (identity diffusion)

Box 2.3 Working with discontinuity in the self

Practice points

- Patients will try to deal with discontinuous aspects of their experience by externalisation (generating the feeling within the therapist)

- The tendency to do this had been established early in childhood, is well established and is not going to be reversed simply by bringing conscious attention to the process—therefore interpretation of it is mostly futile

- In victims of maltreatment, abuse or severe neglect, disowned mental states may include the internalization of a frankly malevolent state of mind. The patient should be given some limited opportunity to create relationships where they involve the other in enactments as their experience is of a hostile/persecutory state that must be got rid of to stop the experience of attack by the self from within

- The degree to which patients engage in that kind of externalization must be carefully controlled as too many regressive enactments will undermine any opportunity for using that relationship to enhance mentalization

---

The interpersonal processes involved in such coercive, manipulative behaviour may feel vital but it is ultimately mostly counterproductive. If the attachment figure responds to such controlling behaviour by, for example, becoming angry and punitive in response to unconscious provocation, s/he is not in an appropriate state to foster the development of the child's mentalizing function. The parent's emotions cloud her reflective capacity. In this way the child's controlling internal working model may further undermine his chances of establishing an agentive self-structure.

A further complication arises if this internalization occurs in the context of an abusive, traumatizing attachment relationship. In these cases what is internalized into the self-structure is a mental state that is explicitly hostile to the child. This can create a state of unbearable tension where the sense of self is threatened from within and the experience of 'badness' is overwhelming. Coercive behaviour (evocatory projective identification) in such cases is felt to be essential for survival.

Failure of mentalization in BPD

The key deficits associated with borderline personality disorder are normally thought to include impulsiveness, difficulty managing emotions and difficulties in relationships (Clarkin *et al.*, 1993; Sanislow *et al.*, 2000). At

---

Box 2.4 Deficts associated with BPD

Practice points

- ◆ The interrelated deficits associated with BPD include
  - • Impulsiveness
  - • Emotion regulation
  - • Relationship problems
  - • Identity formation
- ◆ Problems in mentalization may relate to any or all of these deficits
- ◆ Typical problems associated with BPD may be direct consequences of not perceiving the mental states of other with sufficient accuracy or the re-emergence of non-mentalizing modes of social cognition

---

least the last of these could be associated with a limited ability to perceive mental states in self and other accurately (Fonagy *et al.*, 2000). It may also be linked to problems with differentiating self and other and identity diffusion, which some authors see as central to BPD (Gunderson, 2001; Kernberg, 1987; Livesley, 2003). Difficulties with distinguishing self and other have been demonstrated in analogue studies using film clips (e.g. Arntz and Veen, 2001), affect recognition and alexithymic symptoms (e.g. Sayar *et al.*, 2001) and narratives of childhood experience (Fonagy *et al.*, 1996; Vermote *et al.*, 2003).

Since it is assumed that the prefrontal cortex plays a role in the mediation of theory of mind tasks (Frith and Frith, 2003; Gallagher and Frith, 2003; Nelson *et al.*, 2005), suggestions of prefrontal deficits characterizing BPD (see Gabbard, 2005) may also point to a mentalizing deficit. This is not to say that individuals with borderline pathology struggle with mentalization in all circumstances. However, they do experience difficulties with mentalization when emotionally aroused, particularly in the context of intense attachment relationships. Although the deficit of mentalization characteristic of borderline personality disorder is partial, temporary and relationship-specific, we see it as a core problem.

Arousal and the hyperactivation of the attachment system

Shutting down of mentalization commonly occurs in response to trauma, most commonly attachment trauma. Patients with BPD will sometimes appear to avoid thinking about mental states simply because thinking about the mental states of abusers who are also attachment figures is unbearably painful. Thus maltreated toddlers appear to find it more difficult than other children to learn to use internal state words (Beeghly and Cicchetti, 1994). It is quite likely that high levels of arousal following traumatic experience contribute to suppressing the functioning of the frontal areas of the brain that normally underpin mentalization (Arnsten, 1998; Phelps and LeDoux, 2005).

In borderline personality disorder inhibition of mentalization occurs specifically in the context of intimate attachment relationships. Recent neuroimaging studies by Bartels and Zeki (2000, 2004) have suggested that when the attachment system is activated brain areas associated with social judgements and mentalization are inhibited. It is possible, therefore, not only that trauma-related triggering of arousal may account for the inhibition of mentalization in individuals with BPD but more specifically that the hyperactivation of the attachment system, perhaps as a consequence of maltreatment in an attachment context, suppresses mentalization in these individuals. A number of studies have pointed to the high prevalence of enmeshed, preoccupied attachment associated with BPD (e.g. Nickell *et al.*, 2002; Patrick *et al.*, 1994; Sack *et al.*, 1996).

We propose that there are at least three routes by which mentalization may be suppressed. First, psychological defences may protect the individual from thinking about the mental states of those who harbour malevolent thoughts

---

Box 2.5 Contextual variability of mentalization

Practice points

- The quality of mentalization varies widely in BPD, largely as a function of the patient's interpersonal context
- The clinician should monitor several parameters in relation to the quality of mentalization
  - Level of emotional arousal
  - Intensity of attachment
  - Need to avoid perceived threat from hostile other
- Mentalization is at least in part a function of the prefrontal cortex, and any activity that leads to an inhibition of this part of the brain is likely to lead to the loss of mentalization
  - Hyperactivation of the attachment system
  - High levels of arousal
- Mentalization may be defensively inhibited in specific (traumatogenic) relational contexts

towards him. Second, shifts in brain activity may occur as a consequence of trauma that switch off mentalizing more readily in traumatized individuals. Third, the hyperactivation of the attachment system associated with an experience of lack of safety may drive the individual to seek proximity to an abusive attachment figure. As we have stated above, the failure of mentalizing is problematic not simply because it makes appropriate social relatedness in an attachment context difficult, but also because the reemergence of prementalistic ways of thinking about self and other can lead to powerful complications and profound disturbances which illuminate many symptoms of BPD: the psychic equivalence mode, associated with an inability to employ alternate representations of any situation, or the pretend mode, associated with states of dissociative detachment.

Understanding BPD in terms of the suppression of mentalization model

Common themes

Broadly speaking, borderline phenomena may be understood as occurring at the conjunction of two or more of four forms of deficit (see Box 2.6).

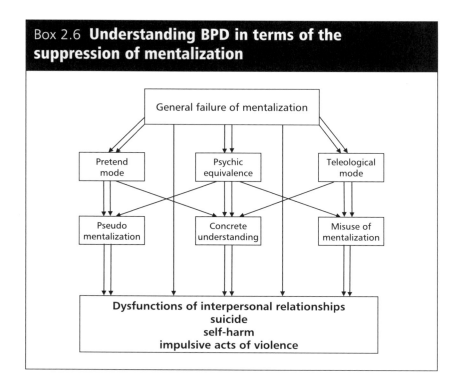

Box 2.6 **Understanding BPD in terms of the suppression of mentalization**

These are the dominance of a psychic equivalent mode of functioning, the re-emergence of the pretend mode, thinking in the teleological mode and the general failure of mentalization. The first three are developmentally early ways of organizing subjectivity revealed by the temporary failure of mentalization. These modes of functioning are assumed by us to generate observable phenomena such as the context dependence of mentalizing, the concrete understanding of mental states, pseudo-mentalizing and the misuse of mentalization. The assessment of these abnormalities will be discussed in Chapter 4. Here we simply aim to describe the characteristic modes of thinking of individuals and how these link phenomena such as self-harm, suicide and violence.

Most readily observable is the failure of symbolization that many describe as the concrete understanding of mental states of individuals with BPD. Rigid inflexible thought processes, inappropriate conviction of being right, extravagant claims of knowing what is on someone else's mind or why certain actions were performed are just some of the hallmarks of the re-emergence of subjectivity in a psychic equivalent mode. Underpinning it is the belief that internal and external reality are equivalent in status. The first formulation to emerge in one's mind is the only possible formulation; it cannot be questioned; no information can be provided that would shift or dislodge that attitude. The affective tone induced by psychic equivalence is commonly characterized by paranoid hostility. This might be an indirect consequence of the conjunction of internal working models dominated by abuse and maltreatment and an inability to question specific states of mind as they arise. The emergence of such paranoid ideation is an indication of the loss of mentalization. As paranoia comes to dominate interaction with another person the fearfulness and hostility that characterize the interaction patterns thus established make it even more difficult to recover mentalization. Genuine grandiosity also occurs in psychic equivalence mode alongside its complement, idealization. In this mode the wish for excellence is experienced as actual excellence. Similarly, wishing one's therapist to be the best in the world in some ways makes it so. It is the lack of any capacity to doubt the accuracy and limits of one's own thinking that plays such a significant role in creating psychological difficulties.

Pretend sometimes carries with it overtones of creativity and productive playfulness. However, when a child feels obliged to tell a complex story of imagined triumph that has no grounding in reality, the listener's subjective experience is one of sadness rather than the thought that this entailed playfulness of any sort. The same limitation arises in connection with the pretend mode functioning of individuals with BPD. The essence of pretend mode is a separation between psychic and physical reality to a point where the

---

Box 2.7 **Psychic equivalence**

Practice points

- Psychic equivalence is characterized by a strong if inappropriate conviction of being right that makes entering into Socratic debates mostly unhelpful

- Patients commonly assume that they know what the therapist is thinking and claiming primacy for introspection (i.e. saying that one knows one's own mind better than the patient) will lead to fruitless debate

- The rigid character of the patient's thoughts are made more aversive by hostile presuppositions of the patient and this may trigger the therapists' ill-advised attempt to 'defend' their position

- Grandiosity and idealization are also expectable consequences of an unquestioning mind

---

connection between the two can no longer be achieved. An adolescent boy's story about imagined sexual conquests that has no grounding in reality will yield to depression if challenged. Similarly, the ideation of individuals with BPD can strain to a mode where physical reality and mental construction are utterly separate. These states of mind are unrelated to creativity although they may attempt to mimic an imaginative, creative process. While the discourse sounds as though it entails mentalizing, the mental states described appear strangely without real implication and bear little resemblance to genuine thinking, feeling, or their combination. We use the term pseudo-mentalizing to describe this type of functioning. At extreme, the patient appears dissociated and communicates from a world from which the listener is completely excluded. Discourse has only the appearance of communication and the interchange is ultimately meaningless. At its most painful this can occur in the context of 'therapy' where the patient's account of an internal world is meaningless and without implication. Internal states and relationships may be discussed at great length but any connection to reality is lost. As such states are relatively stable, psychotherapeutic treatments like this may go on for considerable periods without genuine progress. The absence of meaning frequently generates a search for meaning. The individual who is aware of internal states meaning little may try and find illusory links to physical reality via belief in mysticism, faith healing, spiritualism, occultism and other paranormal phenomena. It is not that any of these activities are inherently lacking in value, but individuals with BPD are not in a good position to make use of them. Ultimately the ideas fail to fill the gap in meaning that they experience and they are forced to move on to another.

Box 2.8 **Pseudo-mentalization**

Practice points

- Challenging pseudo-mentalization in the pretend mode can provoke extreme reactions because of the vacuum it reveals
- Pretend mode pseudo-mentalization denies the therapist's own sense of reality and the therapist can be left feeling excluded and trying harder to connect to the patient's discourse
- The patient's experience of lack of meaningful connection to reality can be the prompt and drive behind the search for connection but the connections found are often random, complex, untestable and confusing—exploration is unproductive

The most developmentally primitive mode of subjectivity that may emerge in severe personality disorder is a teleological mode of functioning, where changes in mental states are assumed to be real only when confirmed by physically observable action contingent upon the patient's wish, belief, feeling or desire. Sometimes the manifestations of teleology merge into concrete understanding and psychic equivalence, but in other instances, particularly in cases where mentalization is misused to control the behaviour of another person, teleology can co-exist with high levels of symbolization in relation to aspects of mental state functioning in the other (see Chapter 4). Placing physical action at the top of a hierarchy of indicators of validity is not uncommon in our society. It is often painful and difficult to appreciate that an attitude implicit in an action is neither understood nor appropriately responded to by BPD patients. Thus a commitment by a psychoanalyst to be available several times a week at an early hour is not experienced as an indicator of commitment. It is taken for granted as a standard template of therapeutic support. It is deviating from this template in accordance with the patient's wishes (giving them the illusion of control) that is experienced as meaningful; special acts such as checking in with patients between sessions, emailing offering weekend appointments, allowing between session contact, etc., are demanded as physical proofs of commitment. The point here is not to criticize therapists who offer protocols of this flexible kind but more to be aware of a constant pressure from borderline patients to show concrete (physical) evidence deviating from a protocol, however flexible. From a perspective of self-regulation, enactments are experienced as emotionally meaningful ways of achieving a degree of internal balance. For example, acts of self-harm may make sense from a teleological perspective, because they can bring about actions on the part of others that represent proofs of concern. This can be mistaken for manipulativeness, resulting in patients being subtly reprimanded. Yet they are forced to provoke visible evidence of concern from others because of their limited capacity to experience concern in circumstances in which others whose mentalizing capacity was intact would not find any reason to doubt it. In some patients this kind of pseudo-manipulative behaviour can co-exist with selective mentalization placed at the service of achieving behavioural control without genuinely considering the impact of that type of control on the subjective experience of the person being manipulated (for example, if the person being manipulated and controlled is a child).

In all these instances, problems arise following a temporary failure of mentalization. The individual is forced into functioning in a psychic equivalent, pretend or teleological mode because they have lost aspects of their capacity to conceive of mental states, either because of a threat (defensively) or because of the intensification of emotional arousal. Thus in trying to understand symptomatic acts such as self-harm, it is crucial to identify the experiences that triggered the loss of mentalization. This will not create a route to recovery of mentalization in every instance, but it will often help the therapist to avoid making a similar error. For example, focusing on the relationship between patient and therapist may intensify the attachment relationship, and as this suppresses the capacity for mentalization it may limit the patient's ability to hear the therapist's comments. An interpretation such as 'You are angry with me' is thus rarely helpful even if it is an accurate statement. If this emotional state did indeed pertain, the patient would not be in a frame of mind where they would be able to validate the accuracy of the therapist's communication. Not only does the comment imply that there is an

Box 2.9 **Teleological mode**

Practice points

- ◆ It is difficult to remember that it is not the action itself that carries most meaning in this mode but the deviation from routine actions that is contingent with the patient's wishes
- ◆ Self-harm, suicide attempts and other dramatic actions tend to bring about contingent change in the behaviour of most people which may be the only route to the patient experiencing a sense of being cared about
- ◆ Misuse of mentalization may be linked to such pseudo-manipulativeness and involve realistic risk of harm to the patient or interactive partner

> ### Box 2.10 **Working to enhance mentalizing function**
>
> **Practice points**
>
> - Therapeutic interventions run the risk of exacerbating rather than reducing the reasons for temporary failures of mentalizing
> - Non-mentalizing interventions tend to place the therapist in the expert role declaring what is on the patients' mind which can be dealt with only by denial or uncritical acceptance
> - To enhance mentalizing the therapist should state clearly how he has arrived at a conclusion about what the patient is thinking or feeling
> - Exploring the antecedents of mentalization failure is sometimes, but by no means invariably, helpful in restoring the patient's ability to think

emotional state that the patient is trying to block out because it is threatening, but the way the therapist communicates his knowledge of this reveals his own limited capacity to mentalize. The therapist cannot know that the patient is angry, as the patient's mind is opaque to the therapist. This non-mentalizing behaviour on the part of the therapist may provoke the patient to feel more aroused and even less understood and less capable of understanding. In general, then, the therapist should focus on the patient's mind from his own perspective, modelling mentalizing rather than flouting its principles. A specific statement such as 'The way you are frowning makes me think that you may be feeling angry about something and I am wondering what that may be about' is a more appropriate mentalizing intervention. Not only does it make clear that the therapist is attempting to understand the patient's behaviour in terms of mental states but also, by engaging the patient in attempting to understand the therapist's mental processes rather than confront unacceptable aspects of his own, it is likely to reduce rather than enhance arousal.

Self-destructive dysfunctional interpersonal relatedness

Difficulties with interpersonal relationships are a key aspect of borderline personality disorder, related to constitutional characteristics of negative affectivity and impulsivity (Gurvits et al., 2000; Paris, 2000; Silk, 2000; Trull et al., 2000) and psychosocial experiences of maltreatment (e.g. Trull, 2001; Zanarini et al., 1997; Zlotnick et al., 2001). The disorganization of interpersonal relationships is often put down to the disorganization of the entire attachment system (Agrawal et al., 2004). However, if we wish to avoid circularity we have to be quite careful not to attribute the chaotic relationships of many individuals with BPD to attachment disorganization, as such relationships serve also as evidence for disorganized attachment.

The relationships formed by individuals with BPD are frequently the consequence of projective identificatory processes. At the simplest level the disorganization of the self structure forces an individual with BPD to manipulate and cajole one or more individuals around them until they behave in a way that enables the patient to feel they no longer own the persecutory, alien part of the self. However, as a consequence the interpersonal world can in this way become a terrifying place, filled with persecutory interpersonal experience. This might explain why individuals with BPD commonly find themselves in situations where they are maltreated or abused by their partner.

Many interpret the association between childhood abuse and maltreatment in adulthood as a reactivation of a particular dyadic template. In our view the evident risk of childhood abuse segueing into adult maltreatment (Briere and Runtz, 1988; Russell, 1986) is not a passive repetition but an orientation of individuals maltreated in childhood towards partners who are more likely to enact intolerable mental states of badness (Cloitre *et al.*, 1997; Gidycz *et al.*, 1995). The dependence that these abused women can feel towards those mal-treating them should not be underestimated. Substitution is inconceivable no matter how destructive or hopeless the relationship might appear from the outside. The characteristic terror of abandonment is a trigger for self-harm and the fact that acts of self-destructiveness can follow the mere suggestion of loss makes more sense if we appreciate that loss means the loss of an opportunity for externalization.

Suicide

Suicidality in BPD is most commonly associated with an experience of the loss of the other. As we have explained, the sense of despair associated with actual or potential loss is not sadness about the loss of the person. It is unlikely that the person functioned in many ways as a genuine attachment figure in the first place. Suicide is a reaction to an anticipated loss of self-cohesion. Suicide attempts are often made when the patient is functioning in the mode of psychic equivalence or pretend. In the psychic equivalent mode a suicidal gesture appears to aim at destroying not the self but the alien part of the self, that which is felt to be the source of badness. In this way, suicidality is on a continuum with other types of self-harm such as self-cutting (Linehan, 1986).

Further, acts of suicide may be characterized by pretend mode functioning in the sense that subjective experience is momentarily decoupled from reality. This enables the individual with BPD to believe that they will survive the suicide attempt while the alien part of the self will be destroyed forever.

Studies of the cognitions of suicide attempters with BPD features confirm our clinical impression that such acts may be committed for the most part in pretend mode. Barbara Stanley and her colleagues (Stanley *et al.*, 2001) reported that these individuals perceived their suicide attempts as less lethal, with greater likelihood of rescue and less certainty of death. It is our clinical impression that suicidal BPD patients frequently experience their suicide attempt as having many features in common with a 'secure base' (Bowlby, 1969); a reunion with a state that can reduce existential fear.

Self-harm

Self-harm exists on a continuum with suicide. It makes little sense without understanding how bad an individual with BPD can feel about themselves. While fleeting negative self-appraisal is a common enough experience for most of us, the same thought in a mode of psychic equivalence can feel annihilating. Individuals can experience a sense of overwhelming badness in a mode of psychic equivalence that can neither be contradicted nor softened. An even more primitive, pre-mentalistic mode of subjectivity, the teleological mode of thinking, leads them to believe that only physically directly evident acts can change subjective states. Following an act of self-harm, the individual often feels relieved and experiences a sense of greater self-coherence. In non-mentalizing, psychic equivalent modes, parts of the body may be considered equivalent to specific mental states that can thus be literally physically removed. The triggers for such acts are potential loss as well as isolation, both situations where the individual loses the opportunity to control his internal states through projective identification. The act itself has little symbolic meaning other than regulating affect dysregulated by loss or the threat of loss.

Impulsive acts of violence

The model we suggest to explain self-harming behaviour is also helpful in accounting for impulsive acts of interpersonal violence. Acts of violence may occur if an attempt at externalisation fails. If the other refuses to be cowed or humiliated into becoming a vehicle for intolerable self-states, the individual with severe personality disorder frequently turns to interpersonal destruction. The trigger for such acts, as Gilligan (1997) evocatively pinpointed, is ego-destructive shame. The absence of the sense of self as an agent that normal mentalizing function assures makes such individuals extremely vulnerable to humiliation. When the person they are with refuses to accept a role of complete passivity, and manifests agency, this constellation may be experienced as humiliating and threatening to a non-mentalizing individual functioning in a psychic equivalent mode. Thus a mere look on the part of the other can trigger a violent reaction if that look suggests anything other than complete subservience. The recovery of mentalization through playfulness can sometimes protect. The destruction of the other through violence is an expression of the hope for destruction of the alien part of the self. It is an act of hope or liberation and is commonly associated with elation and only much later with regret.

Conclusion

The attachment–mentalization framework outlined in Chapter 1 is helpful in providing a developmental model of the emergence of BPD. The key components of the model are: (1) an early disorganization of primary attachment relationships; (2) the consequent enfeeblement of essential social-cognitive capacities further weakening the individual's capacity to create secure relationships with caregivers; (3) the disorganization of the self-structure consequent on disorganized attachment relationships and maltreatment; and (4) liability to temporary failures of mentalization associated with the intensification of attachment and arousal. The failure of mentalization prompts the re-emergence of pre-mentalistic modes of representing subjective states and these, in combination with failed mentalization, generate the common symptoms of BPD. The understanding of these manifestations in terms of limited mentalizing capacities is a useful heuristic because of relatively clear suggestions entailed about both helpful and unhelpful psychotherapeutic approaches to handling the problems.

Chapter 3

Changing views of borderline personality disorder

In this chapter we will consider the changing views of BPD as a severe and enduring personality disorder. Before we begin to discuss treatment it is necessary to understand the longitudinal course of BPD because it is against this background that treatment is applied and can potentially provide great benefit or induce considerable harm. We argue that a focus on mentalization as a core component of treatment provides the best chance of a successful outcome, not only because it addresses the central problem of the patient but also because it reduces the likelihood of causing harm in a group of patients who may be particularly sensitive to psychotherapeutic intervention.

Few areas of psychiatric treatment have seen progress as radical as the field of personality disorder. *Personality Disorder, No Longer a Diagnosis of Exclusion* (Department of Health, 2003), formally marked the end of a sad era during which individuals with a primary diagnosis of personality disorder received inappropriate, inadequate, haphazard, and reluctant care from disorganized services; a haphazard delivery of services undoubtedly made worse by the curious mixture of reasonable and irrational conduct so common in individuals with severe personality disorders which itself generates confusion amongst those working to help them.

The advance in therapeutics and services for PD has been influenced by two developments: (1) the increasing recognition that the disorder has a far more benign course than previously thought; and (2) the emergence of a range of relatively effective and practical psychosocial interventions that appear to accelerate the rate of improvement. Taken together and placed in the context of recent neuro-scientific work, these observations suggest new opportunities for the organization of PD services highlighting both opportunities and risks.

Re-mapping the course of borderline personality disorder

We expect BPD to have an enduring quality. Early follow-up studies even when noting improvement highlighted the inexorable nature of the 'disease', talking of 'burnt out' borderlines, a phrase suggestive less of recovery than a disease process which had run its course, having totally devoured the life force upon which it had been feeding (e.g. Stone, 1990). Therapeutic nihilism was justified by the intensity of emotional pain, the often dramatic self-mutilation, and the seemingly incomprehensible degree of ambivalence of interpersonal relationships. Not surprisingly, in the face of apparently wilful disruption of any attempt at helping, mental health professionals assumed that the condition was resistant to therapeutic help.

Two carefully-designed fully-powered prospective studies have highlighted the inappropriateness of the attitudes which confined individuals with severe PD to the margins of even generous health care systems (Zanarini *et al.*, 2003; Shea *et al.*, 2004). The majority of BPD patients experience a substantial reduction in their symptoms far sooner than previously expected. It transpires that after six years 75% of patients diagnosed with BPD severe enough to be hospitalized achieve remission by standardized diagnostic criteria. It seems that patients with BPD *can* undergo remission—a concept which had heretofore been solely used in the context of Axis I pathology. About 50% remission rate has occurred by four years but the remission is steady (10–15% per year). Recurrences are rare, perhaps no more than 10% over 6 years. This contrasts with the natural course of many Axis I disorders, such as affective disorder, where improvement rates may be somewhat more rapid but recurrences are common. In the Collaborative Depression Study, 30% of the patients had not recovered at one year, 19% at 2 years and 12% at 5 years (Keller *et al.*, 1992).

While improvements of BPD are substantial, it should be noted that it is symptoms such as impulsivity and associated self mutilation and suicidality that show dramatic change, not affective symptoms or social and interpersonal functioning. The dramatic symptoms (self mutilation, suicidality, quasi-psychotic thoughts, often seen as requiring urgent hospitalization) recede but abandonment concerns, sense of emptiness and vulnerability to depression are likely to remain in at least half the patients. When dramatic improvements occur, they sometimes occur quickly, quite often associated with relief from severely stressful situations (Gunderson *et al.*, 2003). It seems that certain comorbidities undermine the likelihood of improvement (Zanarini *et al.*, 2004); the persistence of substance-use disorders decreases the likelihood of remission, suggesting that the latter must be treated.

Changing expectations about the effectiveness of treatment

Dialectical behaviour therapy was the first treatment to challenge the atmosphere of therapeutic nihilism. This imaginative, complex but well-manualized treatment approach captured the imagination of the field. It broke new ground in recommending validation rather than confrontation of the patient's experience, offering skills training to fill the void that generates self-harming and suicidal behaviour, and integrating spirituality (aspects of Zen Buddhism) into a highly potent multi-faceted behavioural treatment protocol. Three randomized controlled trials (Linehan *et al.*, 1991, 2002; Verheul *et al.*, 2003) reported dramatic reductions in suicide attempts. The number of suicide attempts in those treated with DBT decreased to just over 7 compared with over 33 in the treatment as usual control group. When compared with an active control group the benefit of DBT is still evident although less clearly marked. In Linehan's most recent larger-scale RCT both DBT and treatment by non-behavioural therapists (nominated as experts in treating BPD) reduced the number of non-suicidal parasuicidal acts over 18 months. Nevertheless, DBT achieved NNTs of around 4 for suicidal behaviours, use of services and avoiding drop-outs. But, whilst DBT has powerful effects on the management of behavioural problems associated with impulsivity, its effects on mood state and interpersonal functioning are more limited.

A promising evidence base is also available for psychodynamically oriented interventions. An RCT of the treatment of BPD described in this practical guide (Bateman and Fonagy, 1999, 2001) has shown significant and enduring changes in mood states and interpersonal functioning associated with an 18-month stay. The benefits, relative to treatment as usual, were large (NNTs around 2) and were observed to increase during the follow-up period, rather than staying level as with DBT. This may be a hallmark of psychodynamic treatment. Although the effective components of this complex treatment programme remain unclear, the common feature of all the different treatment elements was mentalization. In the study patients received a range of treatments along with group and individual therapy which included psychodrama and other expressive therapies along with some psychoeducation early in treatment. To determine whether the focus on mentalizing is a key component effecting change and to see if a more modest treatment programme may be effective in a less severe group of borderline patients, we are currently undertaking a randomized controlled trial of individual and group psychotherapy alone offered in an out-patient programme. Results are not yet available.

The only head-to-head comparison of psychodynamic and dialectical behaviour therapy was recently reported by the Cornell medical College Group (Clarkin *et al.*, 2004a,b). In what is probably until now the most carefully controlled study of psychotherapy for BPD, they found significant improvements in impulsivity related symptoms as well as mood and interpersonal functioning measures. The trial contrasted transference focused psychotherapy, DBT and supportive psychotherapy. There was significant and equal benefit from all the interventions, although early drop-out rates were higher for DBT than for the other treatments.

Additional non-randomized controlled trials have shown various implementations of psychodynamic, supportive and cognitive behaviour therapies to be somewhat effective (see Bateman and Tyrer, 2004). A possibly important negative finding to emerge from the literature concerns the greater efficacy of briefer periods of hospitalization (Chiesa *et al.*, 2004), the general ineffectiveness of brief suicidal threat motivated hospital admissions (Paris, 2004) and the value of combining inpatient admissions with structured psychotherapeutic interventions (Bohus *et al.*, 2004). Evidence that medication will reduce the risk of suicide or attempted suicide is scarce (Lieb *et al.*, 2004). There is evidence, however, that low dose atypical antipsychotics and SSRIs are helpful in addressing emotional dysregulation, anxiety and impulsive behavioural dyscontrol and might assist in making patients accessible to psychosocial interventions (Tyrer and Bateman, 2004). The trials however usually involve only moderately ill patients and many do not stay on medication for sustained periods.

While it is possible that each of the psychotherapeutic approaches we have considered has its beneficial impact via a unique set of mechanisms, it seems to us far more parsimonious to argue that they all work broadly for the same set of reasons. We suggest that effective approaches to BPD have a number of features in common. These features include: (1) a theoretically coherent treatment approach; (2) engendering an attachment relationship with the patient; (3) a focus on mental states; (4) consistent application over a significant period of time (as opposed to a sub-clinical dose); (5) retaining mental closeness with the patient notwithstanding the patient's explicit attacks on the therapist and apparent wish to push the therapist away; (6) full recognition of the extent of the patient's functional deficits; (7) a highly structured relatively simple-to-deliver treatment package which is robust to the patient's attempts to disrupt the delivery of the package and can be delivered in a consistent and reliable manner; (8) while the package is robust it is not inflexible and is adaptable to the specific needs of individual patients; and (9) the treatment has a relationship focus.

All these approaches are able to present a view of the internal world of the patient which is stable, coherent, can be clearly perceived and may be adopted as the reflective part of the self (the self-image of the patient's mind). In other words, it is possible to argue that all moderately effective current therapies stimulate attachment to the therapist whilst asking the patient to evaluate accuracy of statements concerning mind states in self and others. It is the combination of these two treatment components that is probably most helpful in enabling the person to retain a mentalized understanding of intrapsychic experiences even in the context of a relatively intense relationship. Their effectiveness lies in creating structures that enable balancing of attachment and mentalizing components. Both need attention and careful planning if the treatment is to be delivered as intended given the propensity of the client group to treatment defeating behaviour. Focusing solely on cognition or the environment does not satisfy the patient who feels uniquely vulnerable in intimate inter-personal relationships. Focusing exclusively on such relationships risks aggravating problems of mentalization and undermines the possibility of self-reflection driven change.

The reality of iatrogenic harm

A real puzzle emerges from this brief overview of recent findings on the natural course and treatment outcome of BPD. If, as it seems from the studies cited, a range of well-organized and co-ordinated treatments are effective for BPD, and in any case in the vast majority of cases BPD naturally resolves within six years, how can it be that clinicians across the globe have traditionally agreed about the treatment-resistant character of the disorder? Earlier surveys indicated that 97% of patients with BPD who presented for treatment in the USA received outpatient care from an average of six therapists. An analysis of outcomes measured 2–3 years later suggests that this treatment as usual is at best only marginally effective (see Lieb *et al.*, 2004). How can we square such findings with what we know of potential treatment effects and the new data on the natural course of the disorder?

It seems to us that there is no way to avoid the conclusion that some psychosocial treatments practised currently and perhaps even more commonly in the past, may actually have *impeded* the borderline patient's capacity to recover following the natural course of the disorder and advantageous changes in social circumstances. In Michael Stone's (1990) classic follow-up of patients treated nearly 40 years ago, 66% recovery rate was only achieved in 20 years (four times that reported in more recent studies). Can the nature of the disorder have changed? Can treatments have become that much more effective? Both seem unlikely explanations. The known efficacy of pharmacological agents, new and old, cannot account for this difference (Tyrer and Bateman, 2004); the evidence based psychosocial treatments are not widely available. It is, sadly, far more likely that the apparent improvement in the course of the disorder is accounted for by harmful treatments being less frequently offered. This change is possibly more a consequence of the changing pattern of healthcare, particularly in the United States (Lambert *et al.*, 2004), than a recognition of the possibility of iatrogenic deterioration and an avoidance of damaging side-effects.

Pharmacological studies, as part of the regular scrutiny of side-effects, routinely explore the potential harm which a well-intentioned treatment may cause. In the case of psychosocial treatments we all too readily assume that at worst such treatments are inert (the claim by Hans Eysenck) and that they are unlikely to do harm. This may indeed be the case for most disorders where psychotherapy is used as part of a care plan. There may be particular disorders, however, where psychological therapy represents a significant risk to the patient. Whatever the mechanisms of therapeutic change might be (emotional, cognitive, creation of a coherent narrative, modification of distorted cognitions, emotional experience of a secure base or simply the rekindling of hope), traditional psychotherapeutic approaches depend, for their effectiveness, on the capacity of the individual to consider their experience of their own mental state alongside its re-presentation by the psychotherapist. The appreciation of the difference between one's own experience of one's mind and that presented by another person is a key element. The integration of one's current experience of mind with the alternative view presented by the psychotherapist must be at the foundation of a change process. The capacity to understand behaviour in terms of the associated mental states in self and other (the capacity to mentalize, see Fonagy *et al.*, 2002; Bateman and Fonagy, 2004) is essential for the achievement of this integration. For example, if one's persistent lateness to therapy sessions is interpreted as non-conscious anger or resentment, this may be helpful in that the psychological experience associated with lateness is integrated with the state of mind described by the therapist, creating a broader representation of a hostile state of mind. This now encompasses the passive, lethargic feelings which previously made little sense yet were invariably associated with one's tardiness.

Whilst most of us, without major psychological problems, are in a relatively strong position to make productive use of the alternative perspective presented by the psychological therapist, those individuals who have a very poor appreciation of their own and others' perception of mind are unlikely to be able to derive benefit from traditional (particularly insight-oriented) psychological therapies. We have argued and accumulated some evidence to support this view (Bateman and Fonagy, 2004) that individuals with borderline personality disorder have an impoverished model of their own and others' mental function. They have schematic, rigid and sometimes extreme views, which make them vulnerable to powerful emotional storms and apparently impulsive actions and which create profound problems of behavioural regulation, including affect regulation. The weaker an individual's sense of their own subjectivity, the harder they find it to compare the validity of their own perceptions of the way their mind works with that which a 'mind expert' presents. When presented with a coherent and perhaps even accurate view of mental function in the context of psychotherapy, they are not able to compare the picture offered to them with a self-generated model and may all too often accept uncritically or reject wholesale alternative perspectives.

The problem is compounded by the fact that attachment and mentalization are loosely coupled systems. Whilst mentalization has its roots in the sense of being understood by an attachment figure, it is also more challenging in the context of an attachment relationship (e.g. the relationship with the therapist) for individuals whose problem is fundamentally one of attachment (Gunderson, 1996). Recent intriguing neuro-scientific findings have highlighted how the activation of the attachment system tends temporarily to inhibit or decouple the normal adult's capacity to mentalize (Bartels and Zeki, 2004). Elsewhere we have proposed on the basis of research findings, as well as clinical observation, that individuals with BPD have hyperactive attachment systems as a result of their history and/or biological predisposition (Fonagy and Bateman, in press).

Because of the fragility of their model of their own and others' mental function, and their extreme difficulty with maintaining this model in the context of attachment relationships, the individual with borderline personality disorder may have great difficulty in integrating their self-generated intrinsically emergent experience of their own mind with the representation of it that is offered by another person. A person who has little capacity to discern the subjective state associated with anger cannot benefit from being told that they are feeling angry as this assertion meets nothing that is known or can be integrated. It is either accepted as true or rejected outright, but in neither case is it helpful. The dissonance between the patient's inner experience and the perspective given by the therapist, in the context of feelings of attachment to the therapist, leads to bewilderment which in turn leads to instability as the patient attempts to integrate the different views and experiences. Unsurprisingly, this results in more rather than less mental and behavioural disturbance.

We have argued that patients with BPD are particularly vulnerable to side-effects of psychotherapeutic treatments which activate the attachment system. Yet without activation of this system borderline patients will never develop a capacity to function psychologically in the context of interpersonal relationships which is at the core of their problems. We believe that the recovery of the capacity for mentalization in the context of attachment relationships is a primary objective of all psychosocial treatments for BPD. We suggest that a therapeutic treatment will be effective for patients with severe personality disorder to the extent that it is able to enhance the patient's mentalizing capacities without generating too many negative iatrogenic effects as the attachment system is stimulated. This necessitates carefully designed treatment protocols and focused training.

We suggest that all treatments currently shown to be moderately effective stimulate attachment to the therapist whilst asking the patient to evaluate the accuracy of statements concerning their own mind states and those of others. More effective treatment lies in balancing these components in an increasingly potent manner without inducing serious side-effects. The psychiatrist or other mental health professionals must tread a precarious path between stimulating a patient's attachment and involvement with treatment whilst helping him maintain mentalization. This may be done by encouraging exploration and identification of emotions within multiple contexts, particularly interpersonal ones, and by helping the patient establish meaningful internal representations whilst avoiding premature conscious and unconscious explanations. The principle to follow if iatrogenic effects are to be minimized is to move through 'levels' of intervention from identifying positive mentalizing, through clarification, affect elaboration and judicious confrontation to mentalizing the transference itself without jumping too far ahead. The therapist follows as well as guides, asks as well as answers; there should be no fast forward but rather frame-by-frame progression, pausing frequently to rewind and explore. In subsequent chapters we will attempt to elucidate the aspects of technique that we believe allow patients to develop their own understanding.

Chapter 4

The structure of mentalization-based treatment

The overall aim of MBT is to develop a therapeutic process in which the mind of the patient becomes the focus of treatment. The objective is for the patient to find out more about how he thinks and feels about himself and others, how that dictates his responses to others and how 'errors' in understanding himself and others lead to actions in an attempt to retain stability and to make sense of incomprehensible feelings. The therapist has to ensure that the patient is aware of this goal, that the therapy process itself is not mysterious and that the patient understands the underlying focus of treatment. The mentalizing process can only be developed if the structure of treatment is carefully defined. It is important to remember that the assessment process itself is an intrinsic part of the trajectory of treatment and not something decapitated from the whole treatment process. It forms part of the initial sessions and is a significant aspect of engaging the patient in treatment itself. Because of its importance it is dealt with separately in Chapters 5 and 6.

Trajectory of treatment

There are three main phases to the trajectory of treatment (see Box 4.1). Each phase has a distinct aim and harnesses specific processes. The overall aim of the initial phase is assessment of mentalizing capacities and personality function and engaging the patient in treatment. Specific processes include giving a diagnosis, providing psychoeducation, establishing a hierarchy of therapeutic aims, stabilizing social and behavioural problems, reviewing medication and defining a crisis pathway.

During the middle sessions the aim of all the active therapeutic work is to stimulate an ever-increasing mentalizing ability. The more specific technical aspects of this phase of treatment are discussed in Chapters 8–10. In the final stage preparation is made for ending intensive treatment. This requires the therapist to focus on the feelings of loss associated with ending treatment and how to maintain gains that have been made, as well as developing, in conjunction with the patient, an appropriate follow-up programme tailored to his particular needs—the oft-repeated view by protagonists of particular models of therapy that patients with severe personality disorder improve adequately following 12–18 months of treatment to the extent that they require no further support is fanciful and remains part of research mythology rather than realistic clinical practice.

Initial phase
Assessment of mentalization

This is discussed in detail in Chapter 5.

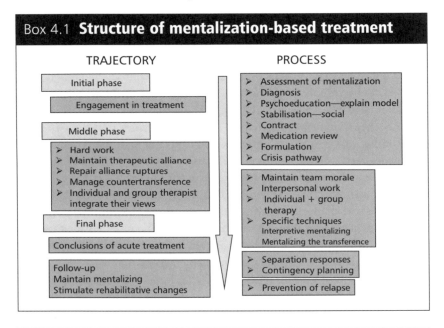

Box 4.1 **Structure of mentalization-based treatment**

TRAJECTORY

PROCESS

Initial phase

Engagement in treatment

Middle phase

➤ Hard work
➤ Maintain therapeutic alliance
➤ Repair alliance ruptures
➤ Manage countertransference
➤ Individual and group therapist integrate their views

Final phase

Conclusions of acute treatment

Follow-up
Maintain mentalizing
Stimulate rehabilitative changes

➤ Assessment of mentalization
➤ Diagnosis
➤ Psychoeducation—explain model
➤ Stabilisation—social
➤ Contract
➤ Medication review
➤ Formulation
➤ Crisis pathway

➤ Maintain team morale
➤ Interpersonal work
➤ Individual + group therapy
➤ Specific techniques
  Interpretive mentalizing
  Mentalizing the transference

➤ Separation responses
➤ Contingency planning

➤ Prevention of relapse

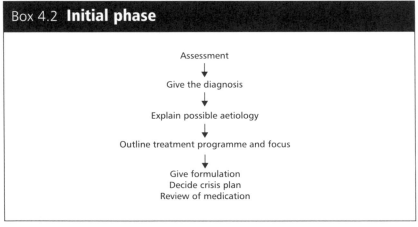

Box 4.2 **Initial phase**

Assessment
↓
Give the diagnosis
↓
Explain possible aetiology
↓
Outline treatment programme and focus
↓
Give formulation
Decide crisis plan
Review of medication

Giving the diagnosis and introducing the approach

Mental health professionals have expressed a great deal of anxiety about giving a patient the diagnosis of personality disorder. Fears are rightly expressed about pejorative overtones, judgmental attitudes, blaming the patient, attacking the very 'soul' of the individual, and stigmatizing the patient for life.

> One of our patients complained that even after treatment, when she no longer met criteria for personality disorder, medical staff treated her with suspicion and uncertainty as soon as they saw her notes, despite her obvious ability to interact with services appropriately.

Despite these potential drawbacks we firmly believe that it is both necessary and constructive to give the patient an appropriate diagnosis. But how does one give the diagnosis in such a way that it is beneficial and helpful? This is less of a problem with patients who show characteristics of non-comorbid borderline personality disorder although even then it may be difficult. But it becomes more difficult if the patient is co-morbid for borderline, narcissistic, paranoid and anti-social personality disorder and also has an Axis-1 disorder. We cannot hide behind the failings of nosology, pass responsibility and blame to inadequate diagnostic systems, or simply say that we do not believe in diagnosis. Even if we do not believe in categorical diagnostic systems someone else in the mental health service is likely to have given the patient a diagnosis or simply to have told the patient that their needs cannot be met within the normal service 'because they have a personality disorder which is untreatable'. Uncertainty and doubt about the value of diagnosis may be appropriate but avoidance and lack of clarity is likely to induce distrust in the patient about the competence of the practitioner and make the development of a therapeutic alliance more difficult.

Let us assume that you are taking a categorical approach to personality and have concluded that the patient has BPD. In our experience the best approach is to be direct and explanatory bearing in mind that you want to stimulate the patient's capacity to reflect on himself and on your perspective about him. There are many ways to go about this and we do not presume to have the correct answer. You, the reader, may have better ways of explaining the diagnosis and, if so, you should keep to what you do. However the primary purpose of giving the diagnosis from the perspective of MBT is to stimulate the patient to consider all aspects of himself and for him to reflect on your thoughts about him whilst you demonstrate your capacity to consider his problems.

When giving the diagnosis it is necessary to frequently check out the patient's understanding of what you are saying. It is anti-mentalizing on your part to make assumptions about how much or how little the patient knows. If you assume too much you will induce defensiveness or, if too little, you will be challenged as patronizing. It is equally anti-mentalizing to 'make sure that the patient has understood what you are saying'. The point is not to 'tell' the patient what you know and to demonstrate the extent of your knowledge but to stimulate reflection. The mentalizing therapist finds out what the patient himself has understood about what he has said. In principle you are trying to find out if what you have in your mind about the patient actually corresponds to a state of mind which he recognises. You are not trying to persuade the patient of your viewpoint.

Opening a 'dialogue about diagnosis'

You may wish to begin with a clear statement of your diagnosis but in general it is best to move towards diagnosis sensitively, asking a patient about what sort of person he feels that he is. Some questions associated with this process are summarized in Box 4.3.

Eventually the diagnosis should be broached:

> 'Trying to put together everything that you have told me I think that you have border-line personality disorder. Have you ever heard of the diagnosis?'

If the patient has some prior knowledge of the disorder then ask what he understands by what he has learnt. More specifically try to access his underlying feelings about talking and thinking about himself 'as having a diagnosis'. For some patients the process may stimulate anxiety whilst for others it is a relief to be told that what has been happening to them over a period of years is well recognized by mental health professionals and part of a known psychological problem. Yet others may find it de-humanizing and demeaning. So the

---

Box 4.3 Establishing a diagnosis

- How would you describe yourself as a person?
- What makes you an individual?
- How would someone else describe you?
- What sort of person are you in close relationships?
- What are your best features as a person?

therapist must ensure that his attitude is thoughtful and sensitive and at times reassuring. In particular, the discussions should be illustrated by relevant examples from the patient's story to exemplify what is actually meant. Judicious use of clinical examples known to the therapist from previous experience may also be useful to relieve pressure by focusing temporarily away from the patient himself.

In our experience, once the diagnosis has been broached in a sensitive manner it becomes less of a philosophical conundrum and more of a stimulus to understand what the underlying problems actually are. This requires a dialogue about our understanding of the development of BPD—giving an explanation—and at this point a conflict arises for the mentalizing therapist. On the one hand it could become anti-mentalizing to promote our understanding of the disorder as an enfeeblement of mentalizing within the context of attachment relationships, and yet on the other hand it is important that the patient understands the mentalizing focus of treatment and our reasons for taking this particular approach.

Giving an explanation

Psychoeducation

Psychoeducation is perfectly in keeping with our model. The therapist explains the possible causes of BPD, the consequential psychological problems and difficulties in maintaining a mentalizing mind, the goals of treatment and how group and individual therapy are used to stabilize mentalizing in the context of attachment relationships. Nevertheless the primary method used to help a patient appreciate the process of therapy is not through 'education' but by engaging him in the work itself during the initial sessions. The therapist listens carefully to the way in which the patient talks about himself and others, identifies features suggestive of mentalizing strengths, highlights emotional competencies and when these positive aspects of mentalizing occur, uses them to explain the therapy process.

> 'You sound like you really understood what happened then. Increasing your ability to do that even when you are upset, hurt or having other feelings is the focus of our work together. In therapy we will come across a lot of experiences that you have, both here and outside, which we won't understand. One of the main tasks of therapy is for us to explore those times so that we can make sense of what might have been going on in your mind at the time'.

An attachment understanding of borderline personality disorder

Our understanding of BPD outlined in Chapter 2 is discussed with patients at the beginning of treatment, initially in the assessment interviews, but this can be followed by a more detailed discussion in the first individual session and in the group.

Patients start therapy with an individual session. This is followed by the first group session which allows the patient to reflect on what the individual therapist has told him and to discuss it with his peer group. The advantage of further discussion in the group is that misunderstandings or questions arising from the individual session can be corrected by the group therapist and explored between the patients themselves.

In discussing the origins of BPD there is a danger of over-simplifying the causes on the one hand and on the other of becoming excessively complicated. Some patients feel patronized if therapists give explanations that appear trite. They react by becoming angry. Others feel overwhelmed by the information. They become perplexed. It is therefore important that the therapist gauges the patient's knowledge and capacity to focus on new concepts carefully before embarking on explanations. In our experience it is becoming increasingly common to find that higher functioning patients have sought information on the internet before coming for treatment and so the therapist should first explore what the patient knows about the disorder—'Maybe you have already read something yourself?' It is essential that 'giving the model' does not mimic a school room in which a teacher imparts information that needs to be learnt by patients. Some individuals will want to treat the exercise like a school lesson, but this commonly indicates that mentalizing has been switched off and teleological functions are in the ascendant. Borderline patients feel cared about according to concrete outcomes so imparting information like a teacher can be converted into a signal indicating 'real' care. For the most part it is best to allow the patient to consider each aspect of the developmental model in terms of his own life and to consider its relevance to him. Rather than giving a long and complicated explanation the therapist should give simple and short accounts of each aspect of the model, preferably in terms of the patient's own history and current problems. The explanation must be tailored to the individual himself to stimulate a reappraisal of his own understanding of his problems and, in the furtherance of mentalizing, each problem area should be linked to the treatment programme.

> **Therapist:** It sounds like you and your Mum just did not see eye to eye and that you felt that she did not really understand things. But you did not give up trying to let her know that you were unhappy. Even when you were a teenager it sounds like you wanted her to recognize that you were in trouble, for example asking her to come to the school when you were expelled and to the hospital when you took an overdose. What is your understanding of why she did not seem to respond?
>
> **Patient:** She was just a horrible woman (a non-mentalizing explanation because of its lack of development)

Therapist: I suspect that it might have been more complicated than that and in the treatment we will help you explore that a bit more. One feature of treatment is that we ask patients to reconsider some of their personal explanations of events and expecially how they understand things now. In the group therapy you have a chance to hear other people's understanding of your problems which will help you reappraise your own understanding.

One possibility is that you will begin to feel that people here do not understand and you must let us know if that is the case. We all bring our past experiences to present situations and you have told me that you have never really trusted anyone so you will be constantly on the look out to see if we understand, so talk to your individual therapist about this and perhaps let the group know if you feel that they are misunderstanding what you are trying to tell them.

Treatment programme

There are two variants of MBT. The first is a day hospital programme in which patients attend initially on a 5-day per week basis. The maximum length of time in this programme is 18–24 months. The second adaptation of MBT is an 18-month intensive out-patient treatment which consists of one individual session of 50 minutes per week, and group session of 90 minutes per week. In both programmes the group therapist is different from the individual therapist.

Entrance to the day hospital programme requires the patient to show at least some of a number of features which include high risk to self or others, inadequate social support, repeated hospital admissions interfering with adaptations to everyday living, unstable housing, substance misuse and fragmented mentalizing. Patients who show some capacity for everyday living and have stable social support and accommodation are more likely to be treated within the intensive out-patient programme, particularly if their mentalizing processes are characterized only by vulnerability in close emotional relationships.

At present there is no agreed measure of severity of personality disorder and so it remains impossible to assign individuals to one programme or the other according to a score on a recognized instrument. The primary considerations are risk and instability of social circumstances. There is little worse than being responsible for the treatment of a patient who is at high risk and having no way of tracing him when he fails to attend appointments because he regularly changes accommodation and has no mobile telephone. Engaging such an individual in the day hospital programme gives him the opportunity to attend throughout the working day rather than at specific hours so, even within his chaos, he is more likely to remain in contact until a therapeutic alliance can be fostered to stabilize attendance.

Day hospital programme

This programme is a combination of individual and group psychotherapy focusing on implicit mentalizing processes and expressive therapies promoting skills in explicit mentalizing.

We are commonly asked for the detail of the programme in terms of the exact structure and content of each group but this is probably the least important aspect of the treatment organization. What is important is the interrelationship of the different aspects of the programme, the working relationship between the different therapists, the continuity of themes between the groups, and the consistency with which the treatment is applied over a period of time. Such non-specific aspects probably form the key to effective treatment and the specificity of the therapeutic activities remains to be determined.

It will come as no surprise to the reader that integration within the programme is achieved through our focus on mentalizing. All groups have an overall aim of increasing mentalizing and within a framework that encourages exploration of minds by minds, even if the route to this goal is via explicit techniques such as artwork and writing.

Details of the programme are included in our original book.

Intensive out-patient programme

Patients are offered one individual session (50 minutes) and one group session (90 minutes) per week. This is not an 'a la carte' menu but a 'fixed' meal and the requirements placed on patients are more onerous than those placed on day hospital patients because participants are less chaotic and have better mentalizing abilities and some capacity for attentional and affective control. We clarify at the outset of treatment that the two aspects of the programme, namely the group and individual sessions, are not divisible and that frequent absence from one leads to discussion about continuation in treatment. It is not our policy to simply discharge someone because of non-attendance. But it is our guiding principle that if someone does not attend one aspect of the programme then this is discussed with him in the next session he attends, whether it is the individual or group session. It is more common for patients to fail attendance at the group than the individual session so non-attendance in the group requires the individual therapist to explore the underlying reasons for absence in the next individual meeting. Only when it appears impossible to help the patient to return to the group is the question of discharge from the programme raised. It is not possible to give an exact point at which this occurs but the patients are told at the beginning of treatment that persistent and prolonged absence from the any aspect of the programme will lead to discharge to our low maintenance out-patient clinic for further consideration of

treatment. Return to the programme remains possible after this but only following further work on the underlying anxieties.

This more rigorous stance about attendance is taken because many patients
find the individual session more acceptable than the group session and attend
the former and not the latter. On occasions this has understandably stimulated
patients and others to ask why we have group sessions at all. 'The group is no
good and I don't get anything out of it' may become the refrain and eventually
the individual therapist is challenged to explain the purpose of the groups.
This question should not be avoided by the therapist but understood from a
perspective of mentalizing with some judicious further explanation about the
importance of the group work. Of course the reason for group therapy should
have already been explained towards the end of the assessment.

Why group work?

Many patients are reluctant to participate in group therapy and their lack of
enthusiasm surfaces as soon as group therapy becomes a reality. The patient
may have apparently accepted the inevitability of group work in the assessment
interviews but secretly only done so to access individual therapy. This must be
addressed as soon as treatment starts. Borderline patients have a reduced
capacity to keep themselves in mind or to recognize that others have them in
mind when listening to the problems of others which accounts, to some degree,
for their anxiety about groups and their oscillations between over- and under-
involvement with others. As they become involved with someone else's problems they lose themselves in their own mind and in the mind of the other and,
when they do so, they begin to feel alone and self-less which in turn leads to
rapid distancing from the other person to save themselves.

You need a convincing reason for group therapy and a way of discussing it
with the patient that does not become patronizing or frightening but is
encouraging and explanatory. It is best if a team can develop their own understanding about the reason for group therapy within a mentalizing framework
so that a consistent explanation is given and is in keeping with the overall
approach.

Many therapists explain group therapy by talking about the ability of people
to function within groups in society and how group therapy can be used to
practise this exceptionally complex skill requiring a high level of mentalizing.
In many ways the capacity to function well within constantly changing social
situations and within social groups is a peculiarly human attribute and many
borderline patients decompensate when the 'going gets tough'. Social interactions create anxiety, misunderstandings abound and mental collapse is
inevitable, often leading to flight or fight. So, to explain group therapy we first

discuss the conscious anxieties the patient has about groups and link them to experiences of the patient when mixing with friends or others in social situations. We try to understand the feelings that the patient has about groups, for example about having to share with others when feeling that they have always been deprived or being concerned that others will not be interested in their problems. But primarily we discuss the power of group therapy to stimulate the capacity of the patient to manage anxiety within highly charged circumstances whilst maintaining mentalizing. It is in the group that patients can truly practise balancing emotional states evoked in a complex situation and their ability to continue mentalizing. The group requires patients to hold themselves in mind whilst trying to understand the mind of a number of others at the same time, which is an essential ability in all relationships.

Here is an explanation (condensed from a whole session) about the reason for group therapy given to a patient. We make no claims that it is a perfect explanation but it does contain the essential components of suggesting that the purpose is to consider one's own mind and the mind of others within a dynamic process:

> Groups are very difficult for all of us but they remain the context in which we lead our lives. All of us meet with other people and have to function in relation to others, sometimes suppressing our feelings and ideas because we know that they may cause offence or lead to reactions that we do not want. Negotiating all this is part of our everyday life. We have to learn how to say things whilst remaining true to ourselves. The purpose of our groups is to work all this out and to learn that we can discuss things, even personal things about ourselves or our feelings for others, without causing negative reactions in others whilst feeling that we have expressed what we mean. This requires us to understand not only our own motives but also to understand the reactions of others to what we are saying. We also need to be able to think about others' responses and to change our own way of thinking accordingly, otherwise we simply insist that others take on our views. One problem we all have is respecting different views. We try to focus on this process in the groups. We hope that if you have a problem discussing things in the group you will be able to talk to your individual therapist about it which will help you feel stronger to talk about it in the group.

Contracts

Clarification of some basic rules and giving guidance

We follow the common 'rules of engagement' that are applied when treating patients with psychotherapy in health services. We have a commitment to implement the treatment programme professionally and with interpersonal respect just as patients have an obligation to attend to their difficulties within the boundary of the treatment outline. There are particular 'rules' about violence and use of drugs and alcohol and guidelines about sexual relationships between patients; that is, they interfere with treatment of both parties. These are discussed in more detail in our description of the programme in the primary manual. The question here is how the therapist explains the 'rules' to the patient.

It is wise to be straightforward about general 'rules' and guidelines, to have a leaflet or information sheet about them and to make them as clear as possible so that they are understandable to both patient and therapist. It is inadequate simply to state 'rules' or to give guidance without giving reasons. A discussion about why they are necessary must take place and be explored with the patient. Some patients will accept the regulations without question, others will apparently agree with them whilst privately ignoring them or at least feeling that they do not apply to them. Others will actively challenge 'rules' seeing them as authoritarian, unenforceable and excessively restrictive. Whatever the reaction, the therapist must discuss the underlying reasons for the recommendations and explore the patients' response. So what are the underlying reasons?

First, there is a general point that anything that reduces mentalizing is antipathetic to the treatment programme. Drugs and alcohol alter and interfere with exploration of mental states and as such negate the overall aim of treatment. Sexual relationships involve 'pairing' of minds which alienates others within the group. Violence controls minds through fear, closing them down rather than opening them up. So, we suggest to the patient that anything that is likely to reduce their interest in the whole group, alienates them from the group, or prevents them reflecting on themselves is not recommended. Second, we explain that there is some overlap between the areas of the brain responsible for mentalizing and those that are affected by drugs and alcohol and even sexual relationships. This surprises many patients, and we have found that the best way to explain this is to point out that when anyone is excited, in love, or smoking cannabis, there is often no space in their minds for others. The person in love does not reflect but becomes preoccupied with their loved one, the person 'high' on cannabis becomes self-centred and may even be in an altered state of consciousness unaware of others around, and the person who is violent or threatening has his mind taken over altogether. Our view about the overlap between the neurobiological systems responsible for addiction and those driving attachment relationships is discussed in more detail elsewhere (see Further reading). Finally we also know from empirical data that improvement in BPD can take place over time but this natural progression can be influenced by such factors as substance misuse which seems to prevent patients taking advantage of felicitous social and interpersonal circumstances and decreases the likelihood of remission. The patient should be made aware of this.

Individual contracts

Rules apply to a whole group, protect the integrity of an overall treatment programme, and define boundaries of professional involvement. Contracts tend
to be individualized and specific, often targeting particular areas likely to
cause problems in treatment. We are not great proponents of contracts.
Fluctuating mentalizing capacity means that a patient who agrees to a contract
at one point may not actually have the same competence in a different context
or have access later to his state of mind when he agreed to the contract. It is
important to remember that effective mentalizing requires a patient to understand his state of mind at any given time, to be able to project himself into the
future and recognize his likely emotional state at that time, to reflect on his
state of mind in the past, and to consider his possible state of mind in many
different contexts. Agreeing to a contract relevant to future time requires all
these capacities; severe borderline patients do not retain these abilities over
time and so can only do one of two things when faced with a contract—they
can agree to the contract without hesitation attributing it with little meaning
and giving it only cursory importance or challenge it as being a further way to
test them and likely to lead to humiliating failure. The hesitant patient who is
wary of agreeing to a contract because he realizes that he may not be able to
fulfill his obligations may well have a higher capacity to mentalize than someone who simply signs straightaway. It is important for the therapist to engage
in this uncertainty and to ensure that the contract does not induce a sense of
failure if it is broken.

There are a number of dangers associated with issuing contracts. Too often
they become punitive and unachievable, and place the therapist in a therapeutic corner with limited flexibility. Therapists often introduce contracts to place
pressure on an individual to control behaviour that interferes with treatment
and we have some sympathy with this view but have found that in severe personality disorder it is of limited effectiveness particularly in improving attendance, and reducing self harm and suicide attempts, which are the commonest
reasons given for issuing contracts. Under these circumstances the patient is
asked to control the very behaviour for which he is seeking treatment and he is
likely to fail. Disorganized behaviour outside treatment is mirrored within
treatment so discharge of a patient who fails to attend consecutive sessions
and preventing early return to treatment simply continues poor engagement
in services. Some patients, particularly those with anti-social and narcissistic
features, may even be triumphant about defeating contractual strictures and
relish their untreatability as they challenge treatment boundaries. Finally, contracts with negative consequences are unenforceable within statutory health
services although of course it is important not to keep offering a treatment

that is manifestly failing. Under these circumstances it is necessary to suggest alternative help.

Formulation

The initial formulation is made by the individual therapist after the first few sessions and after discussion with the treatment team. It is then given in written form to the patient for further consideration. The aims and important aspects of the formulation are outlined in Box 4.4.

If formulations are to be openly discussed, developed and re-developed, the team must be able to work together with honesty and consideration for each other and refrain from excessive competition within the group and rivalry between individuals; each team member must develop the skill of discussing the formulation with patients without over-stimulating their emotional states.

Box 4.4 **Formulation**

- Aims
  - Organize thinking for therapist and patient—see *different minds*
  - Model a mentalizing approach in a formal way—it should not be assumed that the patient can do this (be explicit, concrete, clear and exampled)
  - Model humility about the nature of truth
- Management of risk
  - Analysis of components of risk in intentional terms
  - Avoid over-stimulation through formulation
- Beliefs about the self
  - Relationship of these to specific (varying) internal states
  - Historical aspects placed into context
- Central current concerns in relational terms
  - Challenges that are entailed
- Positive aspects
  - Highlight occasions when mentalization worked and had the effect of improving a situation
- Anticipation for the unfolding of treatment
  - Impact of individual and group therapy

For all patients, reading a frank account of how someone else thinks they may have become who they are evokes considerable turmoil and its significance to the patient should not be underestimated.

> A patient who read her formulation along with the complete medical notes was overwhelmed by the information. On reading the transfer letter from her former psychiatrist and psychotherapist she became upset because former feelings of rejection, which she had experienced when they had talked to her about referring her for specialist treatment, were re-awakened. She felt abandoned and tricked by the transfer of care and that they had not told her the real reasons for referral which were that they could not cope with her and were concerned about her level of risk. In short she believed that the information in the letters suggested that they were frightened of her. There was some merit in this but it was clearly not the complete story. Balancing her feelings of rejection was an appreciation that they had taken great care to document everything that had happened and put in a considerable amount of thought about her. Nevertheless the experience of reading her medical notes followed by the formulation led her to feel overwhelmed and she cut herself despite seeing a member of the team shortly after reading the notes to discuss her reactions.

In the formulation the initial goals should be clearly stated and linked to those aspects of treatment that will enable the patient to attain them. There should be a brief summary of the joint understanding that has developed with a focus on the underlying causes of the patient's problems in terms of mentalizing, their development and their current function. The formulation should also include longer-term goals in terms of the patient's social and interpersonal adjustment which are likely to be important indicators of improved mentalizing. Writing the formulation is one of those tasks that therapists avoid fearing lack of clarity, over-simplification and exposure of the workings of their mind to the critical mind of others.

> *Example of formulation*
> Ms A is 22 years old and has difficulties relating constructively to others and persistent doubts about herself. She has tried to harm herself on a number of occasions and was referred following an overdose of her anti-depressant medication which resulted in admission to the intensive care unit. She has not been able to work over the past year but prior to this was working part-time as a secretary. She is the oldest of 4 children and experienced her mother as strict, rigid and controlling. She was closer to her father who often agreed with her that her mother was a 'difficult woman'. She was sent away to school, in part because of uncontrollable behaviour, where she was bullied and at the age of 8–11 regularly sexually abused by an older boy. She informed the school who did not believe her, but she never told her parents.
>
> She now sees herself as being dependent on others' approval. Without it she rapidly becomes insecure. This applies to many of the relationships she has had in the past which have been characterized by seeking approval to the extent of trying to do what the other person wants even if she herself does not want to do it. This has extended to

her sexual relationships in which she has been abused by two men whose wishes to inflict pain have been gratified by her passive compliance.

Despite these areas of developmental and interpersonal difficulty she managed to complete school and gain a number of higher examinations but when she went to university she found that after a term she could not go back, much to her mother's scorn. She obtained employment as a secretary but this broke down over a year ago for reasons that are unclear. Ms A just woke up one morning and felt that she could not go to work.

Engagement in therapy

Ms A is likely to engage in therapy initially partly because she recognizes that she has problems but also because she will be eager to please and to seek our approval.

It is possible that if she feels that she is not getting adequate recognition or feels that others have not given her enough attention (e.g. not being given enough time in the group) she will suffer in silence initially but then stop coming. The group therapists will try to be alert to this.

Her anxieties in relationships and tendency to engage with others within a passive role may make her vulnerable to exploitation by others. This includes other members of her group and the individual therapist should be aware that this might become an important dynamic within the individual sessions.

Relationship difficulties (individual plus group)

Ms A finds it difficult to make her wishes and desires clear to others and sometimes does not actually know what they are.

She tends to accept that her wishes are those of the other person and she cannot separate the two. Alternatively, in an attempt to establish her own wishes she withdraws.

She recognizes a tendency to devalue others especially when she feels she has failed them in some way. This was explored in the assessment as being a way to manage feelings of rejection.

These solutions are unsatisfactory and she feels angry, misunderstood and neglected although her behaviour becomes passive and accepting of the other person.

Other problem areas (group)

Ms A tries to listen so carefully to others that she tires easily. This may be more apparent in the group sessions when she tries to listen to everybody.

She feels that she has to do something useful for other people and to provide a solution to their problems and this may be represented by becoming the helper in the groups.

Inability to show anger and anxieties in relation to others costs her a lot of energy and adds to her feeling of being tired and listless.

She recognizes that she becomes quiet and withdrawn when feeling excluded and that this has been a long term characteristic. She tends to blame others for this seeing them as 'jerks', 'snobs', etc.

Self-destructive behaviour (individual)

Alcohol and cannabis are used on an intermittent basis but on average 2–3 evenings per week. She tends to wake late after cannabis use or alcohol binges, and this might interfere with therapy and so will need to be a focus of early sessions of individual therapy.

Self-laceration of wrists and thighs occurs on an almost daily basis. Ms A recognizes that this occurs in relation to bewildering feelings with high levels of tension and often when she experiences difficult interactions with others—focus of early sessions of individual therapy. Consider any links with alcohol and cannabis use.

Mentalizing

Concrete mentalizing

Ms A tends to judge people based on what they do and makes assumptions without checking them out. She has not spoken to her current closest friend for 2 weeks because the friend failed to ring her at the pre-arranged time. She feels that it indicated that her friend did not care about her.

If people don't agree with her suggestions about what they should do to solve their problems she believes that they don't like her.

Anti-reflective mentalizing

Disagreement is avoided and she acquiesces to other people's opinions.

Withdraws when difference arises and avoids any conflict.

In the assessment she was aware that she actively avoided certain areas—she often reacted to things by saying 'maybe', 'so whatever' and when this was pointed out she agreed that it usually meant that she did not want to talk about something.

Sensitive mentalizing

Ms A has spent a lot of time thinking about her problems and feels ashamed that she was unable to go back to university after the first term and that she was no longer able to work. She recognizes that this shame is in keeping with her mother's opinion of her as a failure and this causes her tremendous distress.

She is able to understand what is in the mind of others a lot of the time but when she becomes anxious she finds that she loses her clarity of mind and becomes uncertain. Her only way of managing this is to withdraw. She is also aware that she is oversensitive to the opinions of others but does not know what to do about it.

She wants to be able to develop relationships in which she feels there is a mutual sharing and she has found that when she has been able to explain her underlying feelings this has made a difference to the relationships. Although she has not spoken to her closest friend since her failure to phone at the agreed time, she realizes that she is being unforgiving and has left her friend a message.

The written formulation is given to the patient for discussion during the individual session on the basis that the therapist's understanding of the patient is a jointly developed hypothesis about the patient's problems and that this understanding can be influenced by the patient himself leading to a reformulation as additional evidence accumulates. If the patient disagrees with aspects of the formulation it is incumbent on the therapist to consider the reasons for the underlying disagreement and to modify his own opinion accordingly, if appropriate, and to demonstrate that he has done so.

Review and reformulation

All patients in the partial hospital programme and in IOP have a review with the whole treatment team every 3 months. In IOP a similar process occurs. The group therapist, the individual therapist, the psychiatrist and other relevant mental health professionals meet with the patient to discuss progress, problems and other aspects of treatment. Practitioners meeting together jointly with the patient ensures not only that the views of everyone are taken into account and integrated into a coherent set of ideas but also that mentalizing, as manifested through the discussion of the different viewpoints, is modelled as a constructive activity that furthers understanding. These regular reviews lead to a reformulation which can then form the basis of ongoing treatment.

Review of medication

As part of good medical practice all patients should have their medication reviewed on a regular basis. This review can take place in the 'review and reformulation' meeting. Many patients are now referred after prolonged treatment with medications and over 50% are taking combination treatments of anti-psychotics, anti-depressants, mood stabilizers, anxiolytics, and hypnotics. Medication is reviewed at the beginning of treatment but rarely do we immediately change the prescription unless it is obviously dangerous or inappropriate. We suggest that medication is reviewed regularly and only altered by agreement when you know the patient better and he knows you. As a general protocol we follow the guidance on use of medication in BPD issued by the American Psychiatric Association (2001) and provide the patient with information about their recommendations.

Crisis pathways

It is axiomatic that nearly all borderline patients will experience crises during treatment and yet there is no single crisis pathway that fits all patients. What to do in the event of a crisis needs to be documented and agreed with each patient. An outline of a written plan is provided in our main manual. Here we will discuss only the practical aspects of developing a plan. From a mentalizing perspective it is not appropriate to 'give' the patient a plan but more fitting to stimulate identification of a pathway that will help the patient access help when needed in the hope that this will prevent serious self-destructive acts.

Common questions asked by the assessor or individual therapist during the development of a crisis plan include:

> What sorts of things do you feel are likely to cause you so much anxiety and distress that you might want to contact the service? How have you managed those feelings before? What do you feel we could do to help under those circumstances?

Having identified possible interventions, feasibility of implementation over 24 hours, 7 days a week needs to be considered. Many crises will occur in the evenings, at night, or at weekends when the patient feels lonely and even abandoned by the therapist who he believes, if he is able to represent him in his mind, is happily enjoying himself at home with others. Alternatively the patient loses sight of the therapist in his mind altogether and so experiences a painful emptiness that becomes overwhelming:

> 'It seems that you may find it helpful to ring us during office hours but what about at night when things can get lonely and we are not going to be here?'

We insist that patients think about out-of-hours crises especially if they say they cannot think of anything that would help. Their panic is often about the absence of the therapist or team. Under these circumstances there can be no adequate replacement for their actual presence if the patient is functioning in the teleological mode—in this psychological mode the loss of capacity to retain in his mind an image of the therapist as having him in mind can only be remedied by the actual presence of the therapist. The question then becomes how the patient maintains in his mind a live and active therapist even in the absence of the therapist. Failure to understand this aspect of the panic in borderline patients leads to inappropriate use of medication and hospital admission which are often used as 'proxy' carers for the patient's lost relationships. Both responses remove responsibility from the patient for addressing painful affects just was he is trying to find alternative pathways to re-instate an internal soothing state of mind. Some patients find creative ways to re-instate a sense of calm:

> A patient frequently found herself becoming suicidal at weekends and during lonely evenings. The crisis plan involved arranging pre-planned social engagements and developing a 'card game' in which she played her own 'hand' and the 'hand' of the therapist. In doing so she tried to focus her mind on how the therapist would have played had he been present. This card game was something that she had developed herself and whenever she used it she discussed why she had had to do so in the next therapy session and discussed how the game had progressed. The game was therefore included within her crisis plan.

In addition to such patient specific plans, the therapist outlines the emergency system that is available to the patient emphasizing that emergency teams will have access to the crisis plan and will attempt to help the patient manage an acute situation until he is able to discuss the problem with the treatment team on the next working day. The patient and the team then organize an emergency appointment which lasts no more than 30 minutes and is focused entirely on the crisis, how to stabilize the situation if it recurs, and reinstating psychological and behavioural safety for the patient and others. Further work on the crisis should be done within the group and individual sessions.

Middle phase

It is in the middle phase that the hard work for the patient takes place. For the therapist this phase may appear easier because by the time the initial phase has been negotiated many of the crises will have subsided, the level of engagement in treatment will be clear, the patient's motivation may have increased, and the capacity to work within individual and group therapy may be more pronounced. In addition the therapist may have a better understanding of the patient's overall difficulties and so have a more robust image of him in mind whilst the patient has also become aware of the therapist's foibles and way of working.

   Whilst this somewhat rosy picture may be the case for some patients and therapists, for others the treatment trajectory may continue to be disrupted and a primary task of the therapists is to repair ruptures in the therapeutic alliance and to sustain their own and the patient's motivation whilst maintaining a focus on mentalizing. The techniques associated with the middle phase are discussed in Chapters 8–10. Here we will mention the need to develop and to sustain good team morale by building in supervision and paying heed to countertransference responses.

Team morale

Maintaining good team morale is essential to prevent 'burn out' and to minimize inappropriate emotional responses towards patients and to other therapists. It is remarkable how even entering a treatment facility for a short time can reveal the underlying atmosphere and there is considerable evidence that the atmosphere of a unit is instrumental in the effectiveness of interventions and the outcome for patients. Bearing in mind that both the day hospital and intensive out-patient programme involve multiple therapists providing individual and group psychotherapy it is easy to see that problems can arise between therapists and that, if unresolved, they are likely to interfere with implementation of treatment.

   Team morale refers to the overall sense of safety in the team and the prevailing attitude. Positive, hopeful and enthusiastic attitudes are likely to instil similar feelings in patients and stimulate involvement in a therapeutic process. Negative, anxious and hopeless attitudes will fuel despair and mirror many of the inner feelings of the patient who begins to feel that what is inside is now outside; psychic equivalence is confirmed.

Team morale is maintained by ensuring that the focus of treatment for the patient, namely mentalizing, also becomes the heart of the interaction between therapists. The therapists have to be able to practise what they preach and stick to a mentalizing stance when discussing their own viewpoints with each other. Splitting is more frequently described in treatment of borderline patients than most other psychiatric disorders, but it is less often recognized as a problem of the team rather than the patient. Therapists who disagree have to work together towards integration and synthesis. But the interaction of the therapists cannot be left to chance and so case discussion between therapists is built in to the timetable to maintain morale and to ensure that therapists adhere to model.

In the day hospital programme brief team meetings are arranged on a daily basis to discuss clinical issues as they arise within the groups and individual session. The lead for the discussion about the groups is, of course, the group therapist; responsibility for integration of the team perspective in the overall treatment of each patient lies with the individual therapist.

In IOP the individual and group therapist must meet between sessions so that prior to each session, whether it be the individual or group sessions, the therapist knows what has happened in the other treatment session. This is arranged by having a meeting shortly after the group and individual session in which the therapist reports the session. Differences in opinion should be aired and resolved if possible and each therapist should try to understand the perspective of his co-therapist. Inevitably some differences arise and these are discussed in a larger consultation/supervision meeting which occurs once a week. It is here that integration of views takes place and strategies are agreed for use in the group and individual sessions. This ensures that therapists keep to the mentalizing model because in our experience it is easy to be diverted from the model and for therapists to revert to their base technique whether dynamic or cognitive in orientation.

Final phase

It is now known that borderline patients naturally improve over time and that they do so to a greater extent than formerly believed (Zanarini *et al.*, 2003, 2005). But the improvement is primarily in impulsive behaviour and symptoms of affective instability. Superficially this seems to be good news but the

---

Box 4.5 **Goals of final phase**

- Increase patient responsibility and independent functioning
- Facilitate patient negotiation about future, for example, with outside organizations
- Consolidate and enhance social stability
- Collaboratively develop a follow-up treatment plan
- Enhance patient understanding of meaning of ending treatment
- Focus on affective states associated with loss

---

same data suggests that interpersonal and social functioning remains impaired. Complex interpersonal interaction, intricate negotiation of difficult social situations and interaction with systems may be less responsive to treatment. The borderline patient who no longer self-harms may still lead a life severely curtailed by his inability to form constructive relationships with others. Patients remain incapacitated in how they live their lives unless they develop constructive ways of interacting with others. The focus of the final phase is on the interpersonal and social aspects of functioning, as long as the symptomatic and behavioural problems are well controlled, along with integrating and consolidating earlier work. The goals are summarized in Box 4.5.

The final phase starts at the 12-month point when the patient has a further 6-month treatment period. In keeping with the principles of dynamic therapy, we consider the ending of treatment and associated separation responses to be highly significant in consolidation of gains made during therapy. Inadequate negotiation by the patient of the experience of leaving (and incidentally inadequate processing of the ending on the part of the therapist) may provoke in the patient a re-emergence of earlier ways of managing feelings and a concomitant decrease in mentalizing capacities. The consequence is a reduction in social and interpersonal function.

It is important that the therapist maintains an awareness of time throughout the trajectory of treatment. The unconscious is timeless making it easy for both patient and therapist to 'forget' about time when working closely together. It may fall to another member of the team to point out to the therapist that time is passing faster than anticipated and that it is time to raise the issue of ending.

When a therapist mentioned to a patient that they had been in treatment for a year and that there were 6 months left the patient fell silent and eventually responded by saying that he might as well leave now—'I cannot see my feelings changing during that time and so I might as well get it over and done with. What is the point of the next 6 months if finishing is going to be hanging over my head?' The therapist recognized this as a collapse in mentalizing in the face of anxiety exampled by the difficulty the patient had in seeing himself as different in the future. 'It is a bit of a shock isn't it, but I am intrigued that you cannot see yourself or your feelings about our relationship as being any different at that time'. The therapist then explored the patient's immediate shock about only having a further 6 months in treatment and the fears associated with the loss of the therapist.

Entrenchment of negative reactions can be avoided by allowing the patient to take the lead in leaving—setting the date, putting forward his own plans for what he is to do after discharge, negotiating contingency plans—with the therapist judiciously supporting him in his reasonable endeavours such as returning to education, obtaining part-time employment or doing voluntary work.

Follow-up

Responsibility for developing a coherent follow-up programme and for negotiating further treatment is given to the patient and individual therapist. No specific follow-up programme is now routinely offered. Most patients ask for further follow-up which may be a measure of the success of treatment but can equally be a way to avoid finishing treatment and an indicator of our failure to address adequately the anxieties associated with ending. Some patients may have had a 'career' over many years interacting with mental health services; to leave this behind requires a massive change in lifestyle which may not be fully embedded by the end of 18 months. For the severe personality disordered patient who has had many years of failed treatments, multiple hospital admissions and inadequate social stability it is unlikely that they will be able to walk away from services never to return after 18 months, irrespective of success of treatment. Most patients require further support as they adapt to a new life. To refuse appropriate help would 'spoil the ship for a hap'orth of tar'.

The following follow-up programmes are available—group therapy, couple therapy, out-patient maintenance treatment, college/educational counselling associated with return to college, and, rarely, further individual therapy. These treatment programmes are not fully integrated into the specialist treatment programmes because all patients are considered in their own right for follow-up and have to apply for further treatment alongside other patients referred to the department. We attempt to minimize the waiting time for further treatment once the form of further help has been discussed, but there may be a gap between ending the specialist programme and entering the follow-up phase. This is the reality of the provision of treatment in the UK and patients have to adapt to the vagaries of the National Health Service like all other citizens if they are to access treatment, whether psychological or physical, in a constructive manner. Ability to use services appropriately offers obvious benefit to a patient who either may have been refused treatment in the past or failed to have his physical health taken seriously. In addition there is considerable cost-offset to health systems.

Out-patient maintenance mentalization

Many patients choose intermittent follow-up appointments rather than further formal psychotherapy. This is organized within the treatment team. Senior practitioners who have known the patient and who are known to the patient offer individual appointments on a 4–6-weekly basis for 30 minutes. The purpose of these meetings is clearly specified and summarized in Box 4.6.

During follow-up appointments the therapist continues to use mentalizing techniques exploring the underlying mental states of the patient and discussing how understanding themselves and others is leading to resolution of problems, enabling them to reconcile difference, and helping them to manage problematic interpersonal areas and intimate relationships. The follow-up contract is flexible and the patient can request an additional appointment if there is an emotional problem that cannot easily be managed. But in general, the trajectory over follow-up is to increase the time between appointments over a 6-month period to encourage greater patient responsibility. How long a patient is seen in this manner is dependent on the therapist and patient and should be agreed between them. Some patients elect to be discharged relatively early during follow-up on the basis that they may call and request an appointment at any time in the future. We offer this option. Other patients prefer an appointment many months ahead and this provides adequate assurance within their own mind that we continue to have them in mind, giving them greater confidence and self-reliance to negotiate the stresses and strains of everyday life.

Box 4.6 **Goals in follow-up phase**

- Maintain gains in mentalization that have been made
- Stimulate further rehabilitative changes
- Support for return to education or employment
- Negotiation of further interpersonal and social problems

Chapter 5

Assessment of mentalization

Some key principles in the assessment of mentalization

Mentalization is part of the way we are. It is encoded into our language, our interpersonal behaviour. There is massive social scaffolding for mentalization. Most of us often appear to be mentalizing even when we are not actively engaged in thinking about mental states. We do this by using cliches or 'canned' mentalizing language. Mere reference to a feeling or thought does not necessarily mean that the speaker is actively conceiving of that thought or feeling. If I say 'he is angry' I may have in mind the other person's angry facial expression or bodily attitude rather than a contemplation of their mental state as such. Mentalizing is unambiguously present only when it is given as a response to an unanticipated question that calls for a fresh construction involving someone's thoughts or feelings. Thus the assessment of mentalizing has to look beyond the enumeration of mental state words and disregard what is possibly 'canned' and focus on assessing the individual's capacity to rise to mentalizing challenges presented to them in the context of a clinical assessment.

Mentalizing is often context-specific. An individual may be able to mentalize quite well in most interpersonal contexts except where powerful emotions or the activation of attachment related ideas leads to an inability to understand or even pay attention to the feelings of others. Mentalization therefore must be assessed in the context of the relationships in the patient's life that require most mentalization against a background of moderately high levels of affect. Thus the assessment of mentalization and the assessment of the quality of interpersonal relations are closely coupled (see below).

The assessment of mentalization may flounder if the patient's level of collaboration is so poor that the type of mentalization difficulty is hard to identify. However, we consider this type of resistance as a category of failing mentalization that is not uncommon among patients with severe maltreatment histories. When this is not the case the assessment of mentalization may identify one of a number of non-mutually exclusive forms of mentalization failure.

The purpose of assessing the quality of mentalization is two-fold: (1) it can help the therapist create a focus for therapy; and (2) in conjunction with the assessment of interpersonal relationships, it can provide the therapist with particular relational contexts within which problems of mentalization should be addressed in the course of the treatment.

There is no single technique for the assessment of mentalization although a number of approaches will be discussed. Assessment will generally take place in the course of routine history taking.

The comprehensive assessment of mentalization in an inter-personal context

Assessment of mentalization should take place in the course of discussions of the way the patient thinks about his or her interpersonal relationships. The assessment of the interpersonal world provides an ideal context for the assessment of mentalization. Below we describe dimensions of mentalization that should be considered as part of a full clinical assessment. It is obviously not necessary, nor practical, to assess mentalization on all these dimensions at the outset of a treatment. However, familiarity with different types of non-mentalizing is essential for the efficient conduct of MBT (see below). The two assessments, interpersonal and social-cognitive, should be conducted concurrently.

The assessment of interpersonal relationships in MBT is no different from a routine clinical assessment. The clinician is required to identify important current and past relationships and explore these fully. Whilst past relationships are of relevance for MBT, the emphasis is on current important figures in the patient's life. The assessor will avoid linking past to current relationships where similarities between these exist. Just as in the early phases of treatment the past is not presented as the cause of the present (see below), the assessor eschews the causal implications of correlations between past and present.

In exploring the individual's current and past relationships the assessor should explore how relationships and interpersonal experiences relate to the problems that the person presents with. Suicide attempts, self-harm and drug misuse inevitably have an interpersonal context. This interpersonal context is the essential framework for the exploration of mentalization. The representation of the interpersonal events that antedate significant experiences such as episodes of self-harm will give a vivid picture of the quality of mentalization that characterizes an individual's level of functioning. In most individuals a concrete understanding of mental states in self and other will characterize these descriptions (see below). In a minority, pseudo-mentalization (see below) will be more evident. Relatively few will be able to mentalize these interpersonal experiences fully and in these we would assume that the failure of mentalization in which the episode of self-harm is located was partial and context-dependent.

The assessor's task is to characterize each relationship according to four parameters. These are:

- the form of the relationship;
- the interpersonal processes it entails;
- the change the patient desires in the relationship;
- the specific behaviours that these changes might entail.

The assessor should explore how a specific relationship fits into the hierarchy of relationship involvement. This is normally evident from the intensity of emotional investment in the relationship. In highly emotionally-invested relationships the representation of the other person's mental state is closely linked to the representation of the self. This does not mean that the thoughts and feelings of self and other are identical but rather that they are highly contingent on each other. A change in the mental state of the self is highly likely to be associated with a change in the mental state of the other. When two minds are seen by the patient as having exactly the same thoughts and feelings or as perfectly reciprocal, they may consciously treat these minds as separate but they operate as if they are not. In either case, in the subject's mind, self and other are unconsciously assumed to merge (identity diffusion).

From the point of view of developing a treatment strategy, the assessor needs to come to a conclusion about the overall shape of the relationship hierarchy that describes the patient. This is described in greater detail in Chapter 6. Broadly, we distinguish two groups:

- those whose important current and past relationships are conceived of as having mental states highly contingent on that of the self;
- those whose relationship representations suggest little contingency between thoughts and feelings of the patient and important figures in their life.

The former type we label 'centralized', whilst the latter we call 'distributed' (see Chapter 6). The strategy underlying the distributed organization is evidently one of distancing, often creating a sense of isolation and vulnerability. The centralized organization is evidently far more self-focused but may also be much less stable with a number of relationships being experienced in terms of the self, leaving the self vulnerable to confusion and disorganization in the context of these actual relationships.

Both these patterns (centralized and distributed) exist in contrast with normal relational representations where some but not all important current relationships may be considered as highly mental state contingent. More importantly, the normal scheme is flexible. Individuals move in and out from close proximity to greater distance from the self without this affecting the perceived importance of the relationship. The normal individual can permit even highly invested relationships to exist mentally independently from them, accepting that the people they are involved with have thoughts and feelings that are independent of the thoughts and feelings of the self—they are allowed to have their own minds. The normal system is also more flexible developmentally. The relationship with the highest emotional investment changes appropriately with chronological age, moving from parent to peer friendship to sexual partnership to offspring, etc. Whilst the particular individuals change, the map remains stable and balanced with broadly the same number of individuals experienced as close.

Unstructured and structured methods for eliciting material helpful in the assessment of mentalization

An individual will offer a more or less apparently mentalized account of any interpersonal event. Such spontaneous descriptions must not be used as part of an assessment of mentalization. Unless the narrative is created in response to a specific question asked by the therapist emerging spontaneously in patient–therapist discourse, the therapist cannot tell if the explanation offered is not learnt as part of, for example, a previous therapeutic experience or borrowed from an observed discourse but used without genuine understanding. Classically we have used the adult attachment interview as an ideal context for the assessment of mentalization. The AAI has several questions which 'demand' that the interviewees start to reflect on their own mental states or those of others (see Box 5.1 for a list of these questions).

Studying these questions may be useful for the therapist in order to identify the type of questioning that generally yields a meaningful assessment of the person's mentalizing capacity. In general terms, in the course of an interview the assessor is required to identify a domain of moderately intense emotional charge. The most intense levels, for example, probes in relation to experiences of severe abuse or acutely felt painful rejection, are often not helpful because they are likely to overestimate the individual's capacity to mentalize. Moderately charged interactions might involve current conflicts with colleagues, negotiating separation from parents, attempts at arriving at an agreed plan with a partner against the background of conflict. The assessor may wait

Box 5.1 Questions that can reveal quality of mentalization

- You described how your parents were with you, do you have any idea why they acted as they did?
- Do you think what happened to you as a child explains the way you are as an adult?
- Can you think of anything that happened to you as a child that created problems for you?
- As a child did you ever feel that you were not wanted?
- In relation to losses, abuse or other trauma, how did you feel at the time and how have your feelings changed over time?
- How has your relationship with your parents changed since childhood?
- In what important ways have you changed since childhood?

Box 5.2 An example of a situational event

Last night Rachel and I had an argument about whether I was doing enough around the house. She thought I did not do as much as her and I should do more. I said I did as much as my work obligations allow. Rachel got angry and we stopped talking to each other. In the end I agreed to do the shopping from then on. But I ended up feeling furious with her.

for the spontaneous emergence of an interpersonal episode or prompt the patient to produce one. In prompting the patient the following should be borne in mind. The assessment requires a situational event that has a clear starting point, a story or a narrative involving at least one other person and an endpoint. Whilst most such narratives with BPD patients tend to be problematic, there is no reason why a successful event should not be used in the evaluation of mentalization. It is important that the patient at least attempts to describe the event from the point of view of someone who is looking on, although the patient's inability to do this may in itself be the telling part of the assessment. Box 5.2 contains an adequate description of an interpersonal interaction which may form the basis of an assessment.

The kind of questioning that might follow such situational descriptions will attempt to encourage the patient to elaborate on at least four aspects of the narrative: First, asking the patient to describe the thoughts and feelings he/she had in relation to the events in the narrative (in this instance Rachel's challenge, the mutual hostility and the resolution). Second, the interviewer should elicit the patient's ideas about the other person's mental states at the main turning points of the narrative. This task has two foci. First the patient is asked to elaborate on the actual past experience. For example, 'At the time this happened, what did you think about Rachel's thoughts and feelings when she stopped talking?' The second pertains to reflecting upon the reconstructed past. For example, 'What do you now think that Rachel felt and thought when she . . . ?'

Third, the interviewer should quiz patients about how they understand their own actions. This also has an actual past and a reflection aspect. 'What do you recall thinking and feeling that made you stop talking to Rachel?' (actual past). 'Do you think that that was all that was going on in your mind?' (reconstruction aspect).

Fourth, in addition, particularly if the therapist suspects that the mentalization is pseudo rather than genuine (see below), it can be helpful to challenge the patient's capacity to mentalize using a 'counter-factual' follow-up question. This consists of asking the patient to contemplate an idea opposite to the one they were contemplating. Thus, if the patient reports that they believed that Rachel was angry because she wanted to shame the patient into doing more, the therapist can ask, 'what if Rachel did not want to humiliate you at all?' Pseudo-mentalizing is sometimes indicated by an excessively flexible response to counter-factuals, while concrete mentalizing (see below) is revealed by excessive rigidity in the face of this type of challenge.

What does poor mentalizing look like?

While good mentalizing takes just one form, non-mentalizing may be indicated by a wide range of possible manifestations. Box 5.3 lists some typical examples. Some key indicators pertain to the style of the narrative as well as its content and the attitudes implicit in the patient's accounts.

Non-mentalizing is most commonly revealed in the content of the narrative. For example, in preference to talking about mental states, patients might focus on general external factors, social institutions, the physical environment, the government or management rather than the individuals who are involved and whose mental state is pertinent to the narrative. A preoccupation with rules and roles, obligations and responsibilities, as if these were adequate explanations of behaviour rather than created to short-circuit mentalizing, may characterize such narratives. In others, a sparse narrative characterized by a denial of involvement indicates a reluctance to mentalize and look at one's own and others' intentions in a meaningful way.

Box 5.3 **What does non-mentalizing look like?**

- Excessive detail to the exclusion of motivations, feelings or thoughts
- Focus on external social factors, such as the school, the council, the neighbours
- Focus on physical or structural labels (tired, lazy, clever, self-destructive, depressed, short fuse)
- Preoccupation with rules, responsibilities, 'shoulds' and 'should nots'
- Denial of involvement in problem
- Blaming or fault finding
- Expressions of certainty about thoughts or feelings of others

Non-mentalization is also revealed in a bias towards generalizations and labelling. For example, circular attributions are sometimes made in what appear to be explanations of behaviour—most commonly, behaviour is regarded as accounted for by a diagnosis or a personality. For example, 'I blew up at him because I have such a short fuse' or 'I failed at these exams because I am very self-destructive'.

Not all non-mentalizing is identifiable in terms of content. It is also evident in style and at an implicit level. Non-mentalizing style may be excessively sparse or excessively detailed. If it is excessively detailed the patient may describe events in such depth that the narrative obscures the states of mind of the participants, for example by endless side-stories or excessively detailed description of the physical contents.

At an implicit level, poor mentalizing is easy to see but may also be easily overlooked. An individual may express inappropriate certainty about the thoughts and feelings of others, and may speak as if they had no doubt that their model of the mind of another person was the only true perspective. Similarly, a lack of curiosity about motives betrays poor mentalization. In others an attitude of blaming and fault finding indicates a wish to short-cut the genuine possibility of understanding.

What does good mentalization look like?

As we shall see, whilst poor mentalization may be readily categorized into one of several types, good mentalization takes but one form. Here we consider several contexts within which the assessor may note high quality mentalization. The illustrations are self-descriptions but in actual assessment the therapist would be looking for *evidence* of these traits rather than statements claiming such attributes. An easy scoring scheme is provided in the Appendix. The assessor is simply asked to reflect on the interview just conducted and note compelling examples of categories of mentalization, ticking either the strong or weak evidence column as appropriate. Each of the four themes are to be scored.

1. **In relation to other people's thoughts and feelings**
   a. *opaqueness*—acknowledgement in commentary that one often does not know what other people are thinking, yet not being completely puzzled by what happens in the minds of others (e.g. 'What happened with Chris made me realize that we can often misunderstand even our best friends' reactions')
   b. *the absence of paranoia*—not considering the thoughts of others as in themselves a significant threat and having in mind the possibility that minds can be changed (e.g. 'I don't like it when he feels angry but mostly you can cajole him out of it by talking with him about it')
   c. *contemplation and reflection*—a desire to reflect on how others think in a relaxed rather than compulsive manner (e.g. during the interview the person actively contemplates the reasons why someone she knows well behaves as they do)
   d. *perspective-taking*—acceptance that the same thing can look very different from different perspectives based on individual history (e.g. a description of an event that was experienced as a rejection by one person and a genuine attempt made to identify how it came about that they misunderstood it)
   e. a *genuine interest* in other people's thoughts and feelings—not just for their content but also for their style (e.g. the person appears to enjoy talking about why people do things)
   f. *openness to discovery*—the person is naturally reluctant to make assumptions about what others think or feel
   g. *forgiveness*—acceptance of others conditional on understanding their mental states (e.g. the person's anger about something dissipates once they understand why the other person had acted in the way they did)
   h. *predictability*—a general sense that, on the whole, the reactions of others are predictable given knowledge of what they think and feel

2. **Perception of own mental functioning**
   a. *changeability*—an appreciation that one's views of and understanding of others can change in line with changes in oneself

b. *developmental perspective*—understanding that with development one's views of others deepen and become more sophisticated (e.g. the person acknowledges that as they grew up they began to understand their parents' actions better)

c. *realistic scepticism*—a recognition that one's feelings can be confusing

d. *acknowledgement of preconscious function*—a recognition that at any one time one may not be aware of all that one feels, particularly in the context of conflict

e. *conflict*—awareness of having incompatible ideas and feelings

f. *self-inquisitive stance*—a genuine curiosity about one's thoughts and feelings

g. *an interest in difference*—an interest in the ways minds that are unlike the subject's own work, such as a genuine interest in children's minds

h. *awareness of the impact of affect*—insight into how affects can distort one's understanding of oneself or others

3. **Self-representation**

a. *advanced pedagogic and listening skills*—the patient feels that they are able to explain things to others and are experienced by others as being patient and able to listen

b. *autobiographical continuity*—a capacity to remember oneself as a child and evidence the experience of a continuity of ideas

c. *rich internal life*—the person rarely experiences their mind as empty or content-less

4. **General values and attitudes**

a. *tentativeness*—on the whole a lack of absolute certainty about what is right and what is wrong and a preference for complexity and relativism

b. *moderation*—a balanced attitude to most statements about mental states both in regard to oneself and others. This comes from accepting the possibility that one is not in a privileged position either in regard to one's own mental state or that of another person, and sufficient self-monitoring to recognize flaws (e.g. 'I have noticed that sometimes I overreact to things')

Extremely poor mentalization revealed during the assessment process

The response of some individuals to attempts at assessing mentalization may compromise its adequate assessment. In response to probing about mental state attributions the patient may be overtly hostile, actively evasive (e.g. changing the subject or refusing to answer the question) or even show non-verbal reactions such as walking out, starting a telephone conversation in the middle of the assessment, etc. Somewhat less extreme but equally unhelpful responses, from the point of view of an adequate assessment, come from individuals who fail to give adequate elaboration to probes about mental states. To questions about why X might feel in a specific way, the answer 'I don't know' may be accurate but may also communicate 'I don't want to think about it'.

At other times a failure of elaboration is indicated by an absence of integration or complete confusion. A little less pervasive are inappropriate responses such as complete non-sequiturs, gross assumptions about the interviewer's intentions or focusing on the literal meanings of words. We view all these challenges to an adequate assessment of mentalization as responses to the threat that mentalization can represent. Someone whose experience has been traumatic in relation to thinking about thoughts and feelings may understandably resist being forced to think in this way. In all such instances, we code mentalization as 'poor'.

Generalized versus partial difficulties

Non-mentalization is typically relatively easy to identify. The more challenging judgements relate to the extent or degree of concrete understanding or pseudo-mentalization. We consider interpersonal understanding to be severely non-reflective if the problems are generalized and the individual consistently misses mentalizing meanings—for example, if the preferred explanations for interpersonal interactions are consistently seen in physical terms, either in terms of who did what (external) or what physical condition such as illness, tiredness and hunger (internal) explains events. Systematic distortion of emotion awareness is a further indication of generalized difficulties. For example, a patient may react to sadness or anxiety on someone's part as though this indicated aggression. Rigidity of communication and relationship is a further indicator of quite generalized problems, such as an expectation that relationships cannot and will not change and that interactions with particular individuals will always be in a particular 'key'. The manipulative use of specific communications and relationships in general is a further hallmark of generalized difficulties.

By contrast, we talk about mentalization difficulties as partial when breakdown of mentalization occurs around particular thoughts, feelings and situations. Commonly, the ability to mentalize breaks down around the idea of trauma when a patient is reminded of a traumatic situation by a particular person and mentalization becomes difficult or impossible in relation to that person. Linked to this, particular mood states can interact with trauma in

---

Box 5.4 Generalized versus context dependent difficulties in mentalization

Generalized poor mentalization

◆ Consistently misses mentalizing

◆ Interactions consistently seen in physical terms (internal—illness, external—financial constraints)

◆ Systematic distortion of emotion awareness

◆ Rigidity of communication and relationship

◆ Manipulative use of specific communications and relationships

Partial forms of poor mentalizing

◆ Limited to particular thoughts, feelings and situations

◆ Particular mood states can interact with trauma

◆ Chiefly arousal but also depression and even intense attachment

◆ The ability to mentalize breaks down around the idea of trauma

◆ Interactions with particular individuals can disrupt mentalizing

---

some individuals. Thus, depression can make a person's thoughts and feelings about him or herself appear concrete and unmentalized. In general, high arousal and also intense attachment feelings can temporarily lower capacity to mentalize. A fleeting thought of unacceptability or inadequacy can become 'as if' it was objective reality. Interactions with particular individuals may interrupt mentalizing. This could happen in relation to particular topics that arouse emotion. Alternatively, mentalization can fail in relation to a particular individual because they remind the patient of an ambivalently regarded figure.

In assessing mentalization we note in relation to each type of mentalization problem whether the difficulty appears to be generalized or partial (see Box 5.4). In our experience, partial problems are often easier to reverse. This is by no means invariably the case and many partial problems of mentalization are elusive to clinical interventions.

Slow recovery following context-specific failures of mentalization

In the course of therapy patients frequently experience dramatic, temporary failures of mentalization. When a patient screams: 'You are trying to drive me crazy' or 'You hate me', the likelihood is that the thoughts and feelings of the person they are shouting at, or indeed those of bystanders, are no longer clearly perceived. In truth, all of us (not just borderline patients) are capable of such temporary failures. Three factors prevent these lacunae from impacting on our lives, none of which are available to individuals with chronic difficulties in achieving mentalization: (a) a self-correcting mechanism rules out improbable attributions; (b) the brevity of the episode; and (c) perhaps most importantly, the normally corrective response of the other person with whom one is interacting.

None of these mechanisms works adequately for individuals with BPD and context-specific, temporary failures of mentalization can turn into a serious disruption that lasts hours rather than minutes. When we act in an atypical manner, cues from the social context help us to readjust our sense of other people. Individuals with BPD might not have access to this as they are often not able to accurately perceive and attend to the subtle changes in other people's attitudes towards them. As we have seen, they are also less likely or able to test the accuracy of an initial impression. Not only can they often be insensitive to the normalizing social context, but the social context is often less normalizing towards them because their reactions, born of the temporary failure of mentalization, are less typical as far as others are concerned. Finally, as is often pointed out, they find it hard to inhibit impulses and thus limit the duration of an outburst.

In the course of assessment, the therapist may inadvertently trigger such a context-specific failure of mentalization. In many instances, the trigger for this is actually of little apparent relevance. A combination of emotional arousal and the intensification of the attachment relationship is probably sufficient cause. However, the context within which this occurs can be quite important in that it points to issues or themes where the patient is unable to maintain a consistent level of mentalization. Commonly, these contexts concern a particular relationship (i.e. being with a particular person), a particular location where this has happened before, or a particular subject or issue. The relevant aspect of such observations is noting that a particular context may need to be gradually approached as the loss of mentalization clearly undermines the possibility of adequately processing whatever prior experiences are raised by a relationship, a location or a theme.

Pseudo-mentalization

The biggest challenge in recognising mentalization is being able to distinguish it from pseudo-mentalization. In pseudo-mentalization a person's overt consideration of mental states lacks some of the essential features of mentalization outlined above. Thus, pseudo-mentalization may be revealed by a tendency to express absolute certainty without recognizing the inherent uncertainty that knowing someone else's mind entails.

We have linked pseudo-mentalization to 'pretend mode functioning'. This developmentally expectable mode of experiencing one's own mind at 2–3 years of age, is thought to be representational in a very limited sense. The child is capable of representational thought as long as no link between that and external reality is made. Thus, while the child of that age can engage in 'pretend' games or fantasy, they are as yet unable to integrate this experience with physical reality. If challenged about their belief (e.g. that the chair they are pushing around treating as a tank is a tank or is not), their play is disrupted as they are unable as yet to conceive of the mental state of pretending. The adult who is pseudo-mentalizing appears to be capable of conceiving of and even reasoning with mental states but only as long as these have no connection with actual reality.

Genuine mentalization is rarely entirely self-serving. When statements are made about one's own or others' states of mind that are entirely consistent with the individual's self interest or preferences one may suspect pseudo-mentalization. At other times pseudo-mentalization is quite easy to recognize because the statements made about mental states are improbable; based on little evidence, they are likely to be inaccurate and yet they are nevertheless asserted with great confidence.

Most pseudo-mentalizing falls into one of three categories: (a) intrusive; (b) overactive; and (c) destructively inaccurate. This categorization is given as an heuristic to help identify pseudo-mentalizing, not as a way of classifying individuals as the categories tend to overlap.

Intrusive pseudo-mentalization

Intrusive pseudo-mentalization arises when the separateness or opaqueness of minds is not respected. The individuals believe they 'know' how or what another person feels or thinks. Often elements of what is claimed may be accurate and appropriate and it is in subtle differences or changes in emphasis that pseudo-mentalization is revealed. Quite commonly this occurs in the context of relatively intense attachment relationships where the individual who is pseudo-mentalizing expresses what their partner is feeling but extends this beyond a specific context or presents it in an unqualified way. Mostly, mental states are described and elaborated in such richness and complexity that it is most improbable that they could be based on evidence. When challenged as part of an assessment (e.g. 'How do you know that he feels inadequate and rivalrous in relation to you'?), the account becomes clearly non-mentalizing and refers to personality traits or makes unsupportable claims about intuition ('I just know . . .').

Overactive form of pseudo-mentalizing

The overactive form of pseudo-mentalizing is characterized by excessive energy being invested in thinking about how people think or feel. Overactive pseudo-mentalization is an idealization of insight for its own sake. There is little relationship between what is elaborated as a person's internal reality and the genuine concerns of that individual. The person about whom such mentalization is undertaken is most likely not even to be aware of it as using mentalization for improved communication is not part of the motivation for pseudo-mentalization. But even if the person thought about was aware he/she would probably find the thoughts about them confusing and obscure. The pseudo-mentalizing individual may be surprised by this and express frustration about the lack of interest the person shows about the understanding he/she has arrived at. The absence of enthusiasm is unlikely to lead to a questioning of the accuracy or validity of the mentalizing enterprise but to be attributed to resistance or deliberate self-serving denial.

Destructively inaccurate pseudo-mentalization

In essence, both the above categories are strictly speaking 'inaccurate' ways of thinking about someone else's mind. However, often they are plausible even if unlikely to be true. In contrast one type of pseudo-mentalization, destructively inaccurate pseudo-mentalization, is characterized by the denial of objective realities that undermines the subjective experience of the person described. Often such pseudo-mentalization is cast in terms of accusations such as 'you provoked me', 'you were asking me to hit you'. The inaccuracy is in the direction of denying someone's real feelings and replacing them with a false construction. A concerned mother is told by her daughter: 'You would be glad if I were dead'. At the extreme mental state attributions can be quite bizarre: 'You are trying to drive me crazy', 'I think you are in league to try and destroy me'. This type of destructively inaccurate pseudo-mentalization shades into the category of *misuse of mentalization* when the inaccuracy serves the goal of one person using mentalization to control another.

Indications of pseudo-mentalization (see Box 5.5), should be noted in the course of the assessment and looked at in conjunction with the assessment of the overall quality of mentalization. All forms of poor mentalization and pseudo-mentalization may also be context specific. Pseudo-mentalization can occur only in the context of a specific attachment relationship or only in a

Box 5.5 What does pseudo-mentalizing look like?

Intrusive pseudo-mentalization

- Opaqueness of minds is not respected
- Extends knowledge of thoughts and feelings beyond a specific context
- Presents knowledge of thoughts and feelings in an unqualified way
- Presents thoughts and feelings with richness and complexity that is unlikely to be based on evidence
- When challenged defaults to non-mentalizing accounts

Overactive form of pseudo-mentalizing

- Idealization of insight for its own sake
- Thoughts about other felt by them as confusing and obscure

Destructively inaccurate pseudo-mentalization

- Denial of objective realities that undermines the subjective experience
- Cast in terms of accusations
- Denying someone's real feelings and replacing them with a false construction

particular thematic context. In these cases we would consider evidence for pseudo-mentalization to be limited. Such evidence of limited pseudo-mentalization should reduce the overall rating of mentalization by one category. In other words, against some evidence of pseudo-mentalization mentalization scored as 'good' becomes 'moderate'. If evidence for pseudo-mentalization is strong, the assessment of mentalization should be reduced by two categories. In this case 'good' mentalization is to be rated 'poor' and 'very high' mentalization becomes moderate.

Concrete understanding

This is the most common category of poor mentalization. It often reflects a general failure to appreciate internal states. The developmental corollary of concrete understanding is a psychic equivalence mode of experiencing subjectivity. This mode, also typical of 2–3-year-old children, treats mental state experiences in a sense overly seriously. There is no distinction between the status assigned to a thought or a belief and physical reality. Internal is equated with the external. The child's fear of ghosts generates as real an experience as the presence of real ghosts might be expected to. Similarly, in the case of concrete understanding, mental states are deprived of their special status and are treated as if equivalent to the concretely accessible physical world.

The patient fails to make connections between thoughts and feelings on the one hand and actions in self and partner on the other. There is a general lack of attention to the thoughts, feelings and wishes of others. Behaviour is commonly interpreted in terms of the influence of situational or physical constraints rather than feelings and thoughts. Prejudice and other types of generalizations are common as are tautologous and circular explanations of behaviour. Descriptions or categorizations are taken as explanations (e.g. 'He does nothing all day because he is just lazy'). While concrete explanations are mostly incorrect, this is not always the case. However, in these instances, concrete explanations are extended beyond the range within which they are appropriately used. They can be offered at the wrong level of discourse, a mentalized account searching for internal motives is asked for but a physical account is given in response. For example, in explaining a violent outburst the patient might refer to the oppressive character of the room he was in, (poor air-conditioning, overheated), but does not refer to the impact this had on him (felt trapped, suffocated, reminded of being held down as a child when punished, etc.).

There are subtle stylistic indications of concrete mentalizing. The concrete mentalizer will speak in absolute terms: 'you always . . . ', 'you never . . . ', 'you totally . . . ', 'it's always the same, they are all like that (profession)'. Such generalizations short-circuit the need to acquire information about any specific state of mind. There is frequently a blaming or fault-finding quality to concrete mentalization, born similarly out of a reluctance to explore complex mentalistic reasons for events. Obviously such a bias is often, but not invariably, self-serving. Self-blame is also a sign of concrete understanding. Splitting or black and white thinking is a further characteristic of concrete understanding. This is another form of generalization that eschews complexity. Other short-cuts are provided by focusing on unchangeable personal characteristics, such as race, intelligence and cultural background. Burying substance in detail is another stylistic strategy. Excessively long detailed descriptions of the sequence of interpersonal encounters can replace economical mentalistic explanations.

A hallmark of concrete understanding is an apparent absence of flexibility. The limitations of understanding thoughts or feelings makes the individual inflexible, opting for and rigidly sticking to the first reasonable account he/she can find. The natural process of working through a range of possibilities and discarding those that are implausible is simply not accessible. The individual should be thought of as engaged in a constant struggle to relate thoughts and feelings to reality. This in itself is an aversive experience that leads to a deep sense of alienation and a feeling of not being understood. Acting without thinking is not simply a failure of inhibition, it is a failure of a normal mechanism that acts as a buffer between perception and action. Normally, resonance with another's state of mind starts a process of reflection and response selection. In a patient whose understanding of states of mind is extremely concrete, resonance immediately triggers action.

In terms of content, a concrete account often indicates that the person is at a loss when faced with a need to find a mental state-based explanation. They resort to psychologically quite implausible frames of reference—mysticism, star signs, the supernatural, or confused accounts of unconscious interpersonal communication. Commonly a generic reference is made to 'just knowing' or general intuition. Concrete understanding, as the term suggests, is based on appearance. A physical state of affairs is often misinterpreted. A shut door inevitably means rejection. There is a lack of questioning in relation to such interpretations. This is particularly characteristic of concrete understanding. At the more extreme, more generalized end of the spectrum of difficulties, fleeting thoughts that might cross all our minds briefly become established ideas and accepted without question. In this context, preoccupation with grievances and taking revenge may be particularly painful. The unquestioned attribution of malevolent intent supported by the assumption of intrinsic malevolence can trigger ferocious rage.

As we have seen, a range of factors act together to generate these and other indicators of concrete understanding. While the most powerful is the superficial or concrete understanding of behaviour, other consequences of mentalization failure also play a part. For example, difficulties in emotion recognition may send the person off on a wild goose chase of trying to understand the reaction that was not there in the first place, say an angry reaction. The difficulty in observing one's own thoughts and feelings generates obvious problems in recognizing the impact that one's thoughts, feelings and actions have on others. If a person does not know they are feeling angry they may have considerable difficulties in understanding others' reactions to the chronically hostile stance they unknowingly present. Inadequately conceptualizing mental states may lead a person to over-generalize from single instances of expression of intent on the part of others. For example, a modest expression of liking of someone might be distorted by the patient to be heard as feeling deep affection, or even love. The bias is understandable and obviously self-serving. The lack of limitations upon it introduced normally by social cognition requires explanation.

Box 5.6 Concrete understanding

General indicators

- Lack of attention to the thoughts, feelings, and wishes of others
- Influence of situational or physical factors
- Predisposition to massive generalizations and prejudice
- Circular explanations
- Concrete explanations are extended beyond the range within which they are appropriately used

Stylistic indicators

- Speak in absolute terms
- Style of finding fault, blaming or fault finding
- Exaggerated characterizations and black and white thinking
- Attributions in terms of unchangeable personal characteristics
- Unnecessarily detailed descriptions
- Inflexible and rigid sticking to the first reasonable account of behaviour available
- Absence of reflection → resonance immediately triggering action

Typical content of concrete mentalization

- Psychologically quite implausible frames of reference
- Assumptions of motives based on physical appearance
- Thoughts and motives often misinterpreted
- Arbitrarily established ideas accepted without question
- Unquestioned attribution of malevolent intent
- Superficial or concrete understanding of behaviour
- Difficulties in emotion recognition
- Problems in recognizing the impact of one's thoughts, feelings, and actions on others
- Over-generalizing from single instances of expression of intent on the part of others to a general and more extreme state

Misuse of mentalization

A substantial number of individuals with severe personality disorder appear to have an almost excessive capacity to mentalize. This impression is created by the patient's determination to use mentalization to control the behaviour of another individual, often in a manner that is detrimental to them. Mind reading is helpful in enabling the patient to 'press other people's buttons', getting them to react in ways that are advantageous to the patient. The reaction called for is often apparently negative (e.g. manipulating the other so as to elicit anger) but in the broader context can be seen as self-serving (e.g. the patient is in the 'right', vindicated as a victim of the unjustified over-reaction of the person being manipulated). At other times the same person may use their mentalizing abilities to seduce or reassure, anticipating the needs or concerns of the person they are interacting with.

All this might give the impression of someone with extraordinary mentalizing capacities. However, in these individuals the reading of the mind of another person is often at the expense of the capacity to represent their own mental state. There is a massive imbalance between the capacity to mentalize others and see oneself accurately. A further imbalance may be observed between the ability to be sensitive to epistemic states (thoughts, beliefs, knowledge), and emotional states and affective experiences. At the extreme end of this continuum the person may know how someone else feels but cannot resonate with this feeling. This constellation can of course give them apparent freedom to cause distress in others.

The misuse of mentalization needs to be assessed in terms of its severity. At the milder end of this type of problem are individuals who use their understanding of mental states in a detrimental and self-serving way but with only limited intentions to control the mind of the other. Even empathic understanding of the other may be used manipulatively in a self-serving ways. Often, this kind of misuse of mentalizing involves distortions of others' feelings or a misrepresentation of one's own experience. A person's perceived feelings may be exaggerated or distorted. While the experience of not being accurately understood is likely to be aversive, the creation of that sense of being misperceived is not likely to be the aim of the misuse of mentalization. More commonly, there is a manipulative intent relevant to a complex set of social relationships. For example, a parent may overreact to a child's mild sadness and claim that the child is deeply distressed about something in order to cause difficulties for an ex-partner as part of a custody dispute. An ostensibly empathic understanding of the child's 'upset' serves as ammunition in a relationship battle. Very rarely does this form of misusing mentalizing amount to psychological abuse.

Box 5.7 Misuse of mentalization

General indicators

- Using mentalization to control the behaviour of another individual
- Often in a manner that is detrimental to those 'mentalized'
- An apparently almost excessive capacity to mentalize at the expense of the capacity to represent their own mental state
- Knowledge of how someone else feels without being able to resonate with this feeling

Mild end

- Limited intentions to control the mind of the other
- Empathic understanding of the other
- Distortions of others' feelings or a misrepresentation of one's own experience
- Manipulative intent relevant to a complex set of social relationships
- Unlikely to involve psychological abuse

Attempts to induce specific thoughts and feelings in another person

- Use knowledge of others' feelings in a sadistic way
- Inducing guilt, anxiety, shame
- Engendering unwarranted loyalty
- Almost universal in the psychotherapeutic treatment of individuals with BPD

Deliberate undermining of a person's capacity to think

- Most readily achieved by generating arousal
- Invariably aversive
- Physical threats, shouting, abusive language
- Humiliating or threatening humiliation; for example, by suicidal threats

Trauma and maltreatment

- Self-protective shutting-off of mentalization to protect from malevolent intent of attachment figure
- Recreate the vacuous or a panicked state of mind in others
- Traumatogenic misuse of mentalization turned against the self → substance misuse, self-cutting, and dissociation

A more complex set of problems arises when there is an apparent attempt to induce specific thoughts and feelings in another person. At the extreme there are antisocial individuals who use knowledge of others' feelings in a sadistic way. This kind of manipulation is characteristic of so-called psychopaths who may use mentalizing capacities to engender trust in order to be able to exploit an interpersonal relationship fully. This type of elaborate control of someone's behaviour is rare. More commonly, the misuse of mentalization involves inducing guilt, anxiety, shame, or indeed engendering unwarranted loyalty as part of establishing control over the other person. This type of misuse of mentalization is quite common, almost universal in the psychotherapeutic treatment of individuals with BPD whereby the therapist is induced to experience mental states that are the patient's own.

A special form of this coercive misuse is a deliberate undermining of a person's capacity to think. Often for someone with an enfeebled mentalizing capacity the presence of another person who is capable of thought may be deeply threatening. There are relatively easy ways of undermining mentalization, most readily by generating arousal. These are invariably aversive experiences for the 'victim'. Physical threats, shouting, abusive language, or just over-taxing the listener's attentional capacities may all serve to block mentalization. More subtly, patients may induce a failure of mentalization by humiliating or threatening humiliation. For example, suicidal threats by a patient may create anxiety in a therapist as well as imply professional failure (shame) and thus serve to partially or fully arrest the therapist's capacity to adequately contemplate the mental state of the patient.

A further special issue concerning the misuse of mentalization relates to trauma and maltreatment. Children often respond to an abusive adult's frankly hostile intent towards them by inhibiting their capacity to think about mental states: contemplating their abuser's state of mind (often an attachment figure) is often simply too painful. Not surprisingly, exploring the issue of trauma in adult survivors of maltreatment frequently generates a loss of mentalization (see above). More pertinent in this context is the need of traumatized individuals to recreate a vacuous or a panicked state of mind in others around them in order to relieve themselves of such unbearably painful states. The traumatogenic misuse of mentalization may even more frequently be turned against the self. Stopping oneself from thinking may be achieved in a range of ways including substance misuse, self harm, or seeking an extreme version of pretend mode functioning in a state of dissociation.

Conclusion

The assessment of mentalization should fulfil the following aims: (1) provide a map of important interpersonal relationships and their connections to key problem behaviours; (2) assess in these contexts the optimal quality of mentalization; (3) delineate significant attempts at undermining mentalization; (4) assess whether difficulties in mentalization are generalized or partial and (5) in either case assess whether pseudo-mentalization or concrete understanding predominates; and (6) any tendency for the misuse of mentalization needs to be considered separately.

Chapter 6

Assessment of interpersonal and relational world

It is important to assess the predominant style and quality of relationships a patient develops using a time frame of at least 5 years. Many patients show a distinct pattern and the therapist needs to identify this early in the assessment process. We have already discussed in Chapter 5 the importance of assessing mentalizing capacity within the context of current relationship styles. Here we discuss how the pattern of relationships will not only inform the types of interventions used but also indicate the form of the relationship which is likely to develop between the patient, the therapist and the treatment team. Remember, characteristics of previous and current relationships should correlate with your assessment of mentalizing ability. If you find a discrepancy during assessment between the pattern of relationships and your assessment of mentalizing you should probe more carefully.

Once a pattern is identified you should point out to the patient that perhaps this will be repeated within the treatment itself—'You sound like you have found that all your relationships become problematic after a few months and you begin to feel unwanted. Perhaps we are going to have to look out for that in our relationship when we begin treatment'. This is a typical 'transference tracer' (see p 134) and is a very common form of intervention in MBT.

Patterns of relationships

For practical purposes we have defined two types of distinct relationship patterns commonly identified in patients with BPD. The first is the centralized pattern and the second is the distributed type. Inevitably, dividing patterns of relationships into two distinct categories is not only embarrassingly schematic but also grossly over-simplified. Nonetheless the aim is to help the therapist to orientate himself to the experience of the patient and to help him choose appropriate interventions. In order to define the centralized and distributed relationship we assume that there is a normal pattern but again we are being schematic.

Normal

A 'normal' pattern of relationships shows selectivity, flexibility and stability over time.

Individuals form a variety of relationships ranging from intimate to distant which together form part of a coherent interpersonal world. The relationships may vary over time and move from intimacy to greater distance or from distance to closeness according to circumstance or choice but a sense of constancy is portrayed. The core self is never threatened. This pattern is represented diagrammatically in Box 6.2.

A normal pattern correlates with secure attachment and is marked by a relatively good capacity to mentalize and to generate coherent narratives of even turbulent interpersonal episodes. Individuals value attachment relationships, coherently integrate memories into a meaningful narrative

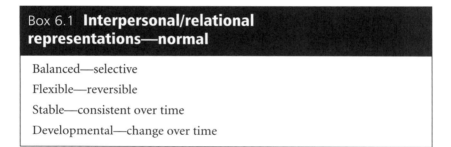

Box 6.1 **Interpersonal/relational representations—normal**

Balanced—selective

Flexible—reversible

Stable—consistent over time

Developmental—change over time

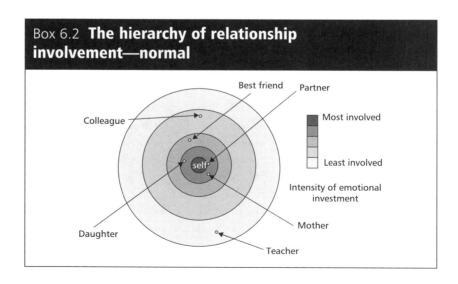

Box 6.2 **The hierarchy of relationship involvement—normal**

and regard them as formative over time. They anticipate influencing others and being changed by them. They remain organized when under stress, show stability in emotional response and communicate negative emotions constructively. This perfect pattern is of course rare! In essence these individuals allow others with whom they have a highly invested relationship to have their own mind.

Remember, these characteristics of previous and current relationships should correlate with a robust ability to mentalize. If you find a discrepancy during assessment between the pattern of relationships and your assessment of mentalization you should probe more carefully.

Centralized

Patients demonstrating a centralized pattern of relationships describe unstable and inflexible interactions (see Box 6.3). Their representation of the other person's mental state is closely linked to their representation of self. This does not mean that the thoughts and feelings of self and other are identical but rather that they are highly contingent on each other. Change in the other person is anticipated in response to change in the feelings of the self and if it does not occur or the other indicates independence of mind, panic and confusion occurs. The key to defining this type of relationship organization is finding that relationships fluctuate between being close and over-involved and being remote and denigrated. The patient is self-focused. Emotions surrounding relationships are powerful, fluctuating and compelling. People quickly become 'best friends', 'lovers', 'enemies' and 'betrayers'. The dialogue contains statements like 'I cannot live without him' or 'she betrayed me', and 'he is out of my life forever'. Interactions swing wildly from intimacy to distance or

---

Box 6.3 Interpersonal/relational representations in BPD

- ◆ Centralized
  - ○ Unstable
  - ○ Self-focused
  - ○ Inflexible
- ◆ Distributed
  - ○ Stable
  - ○ Distancing
  - ○ Inflexible

become turbulent following apparently small slights. The other person is often experienced as being unreliable or inconsistent and failing to demonstrate love adequately. Experience of disloyalty and abandonment is common and the quality of the relationship is often represented in a schematic way, especially when the core self is threatened. Descriptions become polarized with blame apportioned liberally. Not surprisingly the strength of emotion surrounding this pattern of relationship leads to impulsivity and suicide attempts or self-harm, often in the context of emotional turmoil. This pattern is represented diagrammatically in Box 6.4.

The centralized pattern of relationships links with insecure attachment. On numerous measures of adult attachment, patients with BPD are identified as insecure, preoccupied and fearful in their relationships. They have a specific type of disorganized, anxious, preoccupied attachment focused around an approach avoidance dilemma where the attachment figure is simultaneously perceived as a source of threat and a secure base. Gunderson carefully described typical patterns of borderline dysfunction in terms of exaggerated reactions of the insecurely attached infant, for example, clinging, fearfulness about dependency needs, terror of abandonment, constant monitoring of the proximity of the caregiver and deep ambivalence and fearfulness of close relationships. This is the centralized borderline patient.

The centralized borderline patient will not be able to maintain mentalizing normally in the context of attachment relationships. Separation of minds becomes impossible and this leads to confusion of what is within and what is

Box 6.4 The hierarchy of relationship involvement—centralized—unstable

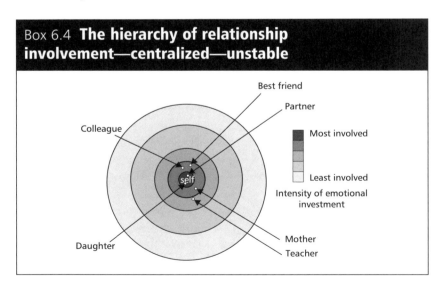

without, whose feeling is whose, and what is self and what is other. The hyper-responsiveness of the attachment system, perhaps related to traumatic or other early experiences or genetic predisposition, has an unusually negative impact upon mentalizing. So, once again, your assessment of the relationship pattern should correlate with your assessment of mentalization. More specifically, capacity for mentalization may be reasonable outside close interpersonal interactions but once embroiled within a relationship the patient's capacity is likely to be significantly diminished.

Practice point

As soon as you stimulate the attachment relationship in treatment the patient's mental capacities will rapidly decrease, making it difficult for him to understand complex interventions. Under these circumstances you must alter your interventions, making them simple and understandable, to ensure that the patient does not become over-aroused which will further reduce his capacities (see p 18).

Distributed

In contrast to the instability of centralized relationships the distributed pattern demonstrates fragile stability (see Box 6.3). This is linked to a detached attachment pattern. People are distanced; there is little flexibility in the system with no one being allowed to become close. A clear separation of one's own mind and the other's mind is maintained. Intimacy is dangerous—as one patient said 'I don't do relationships anymore. That way I feel OK'.

Patients may present at assessment with pseudo-mentalization (see p 72) and can rapidly engage in conversation with the therapist using pretend mode (see p 73). They give plausible explanations for their problems and the insight-oriented therapist may be left wondering what more he can offer. The picture of isolation and distancing may have emerged over time because repeated attempts to have relationships have resulted in failure. Eventually patients give up and, in despair, retreat from emotions and interactions with others just as they may have done from their family. This is represented diagrammatically in Box 6.5.

Nonetheless they can find this 'dissociated' state painful and at times attempt to remedy the situation by seeking out others only to find that this leaves them feeling inadequate and foolish once again. Disappointed, they seek help but either leave quickly when they realize that treatment means having an emotional involvement or alternatively maintain treatment but hold the therapist and others at a distance.

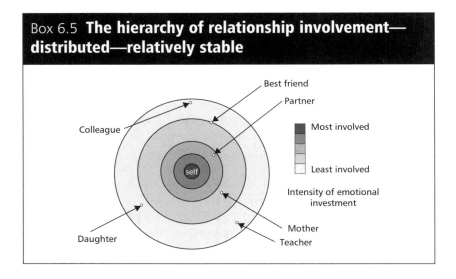

Box 6.5 **The hierarchy of relationship involvement— distributed—relatively stable**

In general these patients have decoupled their capacity to deal with their own or others' mental states comprehensively, particularly in an attachment context, but this leaves them isolated and alone. Beginning relationships or starting treatment becomes a way of placing aspects of themselves outside. This stabilizes their fragile sense of self and once the externalization is achieved, the patient has no interest in the relationship with the therapist and may in fact wish to repudiate it totally. At these moments the therapist may feel abandoned and some instances of boundary violations may be related to the therapist's difficulty in coping with the implicit rejection which the patient's wish to distance themselves from a disowned part of their mind entails.

Practice point

Dynamic therapists tend to interpret what they believe is the representation of a self-object dyad which is being enacted within the therapeutic encounter but we recommend that this is not done at this point. Remember that when the patient rejects some aspect of treatment it may be because they fear that the externalized aspects are being forced back into them. Focusing the patient's attention at these moments on the relationship may be felt by them as undermining their attempts at separating from the disowned part of themselves and consequently can be counterproductive, leading the patient to prematurely terminate the treatment. It is better to gradually ease the patient towards exploring the relationship by placing yourself within the relationship in an overt way—'I think that I must be doing something that makes you nervous. Can you identify what it is?' (see Chapter 8 for fuller discussion).

Why assess the pattern of relationship?

There are two main reasons for assessing the pattern of the relationship. First, it indicates the relational contexts in which problems in mentalizing will occur and need to be addressed. Second, it enables the therapist to position himself in relation to the patient. In the centralized patient the therapist needs to maintain a careful balance between closeness and distance. When the patient pushes the therapist away the therapist needs to push back into the relationship. When the patient becomes entangled emotionally with the therapist, appropriate distancing is necessary. The danger for the therapist is of becoming too involved or too distant and oscillating between the two poles.

In the distributed patient the therapist must try gently to bring the patient closer into contact with his emotions especially in relation to the patient/therapist interaction. The danger for the therapist is of becoming too distant, allowing the patient to remain detached through intellectualisation or stimulating 'pretend mode' through rational, emotionless, exploration of relationships.

Current and past relationships

Establishing the pattern of relationships requires the therapist to elicit the details of all important present and past relationships but with an emphasis on current and recent involvement with others (see Box 6.6).

Each notable relationship should be explored from beginning to end, its trajectory charted and its effect on the patient's emotional state identified.

Box 6.6 Identify all important current and past relationships

- ◆ Characterize each relationship according to
  - Form
  - Process
  - Change
  - Behaviour
- ◆ Explore how relationships relate to problems; for example, suicide attempts, self-harm, drug misuse
- ◆ Link past to current relationships (BUT eschew causality) where similarities exist—'that sounds just like you felt with your present partner'
- ◆ Identify priorities/hierarchy for intervention

In particular the interaction between relationships and suicide attempts, self-harm and impulsive behaviour should be explored. Insist on discussing the quality of interaction, obvious moments of change in the relationship and characteristic interactions. The information will be important as you seek to understand the experience of the patient. Do not simply seek out negative and problematic areas of relationships but give equal importance to aspects that give the patient security, pleasure and moments of happiness. Few relationships are solely negative.

An important aspect of all psychotherapy is to help patients develop a narrative of themselves in relation to others in terms of past experience and current understanding. You should make obvious links between past and current relationships—'that sounds just like how you felt with your present partner'—but in doing this it is important to eschew causality. MBT does not seek to explain present problems as repetitions of the past, and attempting to offer such explanations early in treatment is likely to make the patient feel that their current difficulties lack substance. Mentalizing is not explanation and insight but a capacity to make and break story lines according to new experience and reflection. Rigid adherence to a narrative is anti-mentalizing as it disallows construction and re-construction of an autobiographical story and prevents re-appraisal within a new context.

As part of the assessment the therapist should elicit a detailed account of at least one, and preferably three or more, important current interpersonal interactions in which the attachment relationship has been emotionally activated; for example, an argument with a partner (see Box 6.7).

Box 6.7 **Assess current emotional interactions**

- Identify common communication difficulties
- Explore any open conflict associated with affect storm—outcome
- Characterize ambiguous, indirect non-verbal communication
- Delineate incorrect assumptions; that is, that one has communicated or that one has understood
- Identify silent closing off communication and repetitive statements— 'I know that I am no good'
- Identify faulty communication by listening for the assumptions that the patient makes about other's thoughts or feelings including in therapy dialogue

The patient needs to begin to grasp the idea that interpersonal events are complex, cannot easily be explained and are too easily dismissed as a way of managing disturbing and destabilizing feelings. All too often patients fail to mentalize events even after an emotional storm has passed, preferring to forget about them or to pretend that they did not happen. (see Box 6.8).

MBT requires the patient to focus carefully on their internal experience and state of mind at the time. But importantly MBT also asks the patient to focus on the other person's mind. This means that the therapist has to identify misunderstandings in relationships, define ambiguous, indirect non-verbal communication and delineate incorrect assumptions—'What was it that made you behave like that at that moment? Why do you think that he said that? How do you explain his behaviour towards you'. When we talk to people we assume that they have understood what we are saying and why we are saying it. In fact their perceptions of our motivations may differ from our own and so the interaction gradually becomes distorted. The vulnerable mentalizing capacity of the borderline patient makes this a common event. If it occurs during the assessment the therapist should alight on it and identify the process leading to progressive confusion.

Patients may use silence, closing off communications and repetitive statements—'I know that I am no good'; 'it is all my fault'. The therapist should ensure that if closure statements occur during the assessment they

---

Box 6.8 **Common assessment questions**

- ◆ Questions
    - ◆ Looking back, can you think a bit about what made her behave like that?
    - ◆ How do you explain his action?
    - ◆ Is that something that has happened before?
    - ◆ Is there any other explanation?
    - ◆ What do other people think about it?
- ◆ Probes
    - ◆ I can see that you must have wanted to end the relationship but somehow you stuck it out. Tell me what made you carry on.
    - ◆ You must have been so excited when the relationship started and felt so let down when he was unreliable. How did you manage those feelings?

highlight the effect these have on further consideration of the topic. If at all possible identify flawed communication by listening for the assumptions that the patient makes about others' thoughts or feelings including your own. Many patients will insist that you do not understand because you have not experienced what they have—'how can you understand? You weren't abused like I was'—and yet they have no way of knowing whether you have or have not experienced similar events or feelings. This is not a cue to tell them about yourself but is a moment to challenge their assumptions about you and to question whether they make similar assumptions about others and act on those assumptions (see stop and stand, p 126).

Chapter 7

Therapist stance

Mentalizing in psychotherapy is a process of joint attention in which the patient's mental states are the object of scrutiny. The mentalizing therapist continually constructs and reconstructs an image of the patient in his mind to help the patient to apprehend what he feels and why he experiences what he does. The patient has to find himself in the mind of the therapist and, equally, the therapist has to understand himself in the mind of the patient if the two together are to develop a mentalizing process. Both have to experience a mind being changed by a mind.

Whilst this process sounds rarefied, in practice it is not. You, the therapist, must ensure that your primary concern is the patient's state of mind and not his behaviour. Your principal interest is in what is happening in his mind now, not what was happening then, and your curiosity is about what you or your patient has or might have had in mind which has created the current situation, recognizing that neither you nor your patient experiences an interaction other than impressionistically. This requires you to monitor your own mind as much as that of the patient's and to keep an eye on your occasional enactments, however small. Despite our contention that borderline patients have a reduced capacity to monitor the minds of others accurately, they can be very sensitive to some underlying motives of others and may pick up, with remarkable and sometimes uncomfortable accuracy, your mistakes and weaknesses. So, as we will see, appropriate humility and capacity to learn on the therapist's part is an important part of treatment.

In an attempt to capture the therapist stance which gives the best chance of achieving mentalizing goals, we have defined a mentalizing, inquisitive or not-knowing stance.

Mentalizing or not-knowing stance

The mentalizing or not-knowing stance (see Box 7.1) is not synonymous with having no knowledge. The term is an attempt to capture a sense that mental states are opaque, and that the therapist can have no more idea of what is in the patient's mind than the patient himself and, in fact,

---

Box 7.1 Mentalizing stance

- Mentalizing in psychotherapy is a process of joint attention in which the patient's mental states are the object of attention
- The therapist continually constructs and reconstructs an image of the patient, to help the patient to apprehend what he feels
- Neither therapist nor patient experiences interactions other than impressionistically
- Differences are identified
- Acceptance of different perspectives
- Active questioning

Box 7.2 Active questioning

- Why do you think that he said that?
- I wonder if that was related to the group yesterday?
- Perhaps you felt that I was judging you?
- What do you make of her suicidal feeling (in the group)?
- Why do you think that he behaved towards you as he did?
- What do you make of what has happened?

---

probably will have a lot less. Your position is one in which you attempt to demonstrate a willingness to find out about your patient, what makes him 'tick', how he feels, and the reasons for his underlying problems. To do this you need to become an active questioning therapist (see Box 7.2) discouraging excessive free association by the patient in favour of detailed monitoring and understanding of the interpersonal processes and how they relate to the patient's mental states. When you take a different perspective to the patient this should be verbalized and explored in relation to the patient's alternative perspective with no assumption being made about whose viewpoint has greater validity (see Box 7.3). The task is to determine the mental processes which have led to alternative viewpoints and to consider each perspective in relation to the other, accepting that diverse outlooks may be acceptable. Where differences are clear and cannot

Box 7.3 **Highlighting alternative perspectives**

- ◆ I saw it as a way to control yourself rather than to attack me (patient explanation); can you think about that for a moment
- ◆ You seem to think that I don't like you and yet I am not sure what makes you think that
- ◆ Just as you distrusted everyone around you because you couldn't predict how they would respond, you are now suspicious of me
- ◆ You have to see me as critical so that you can feel vindicated in your dismissal of what I say

initially be resolved, this should be identified, stated and accepted until resolution seems possible.

The activity of the questioning therapist is illustrated in the following vignette.

The disappointed patient

Patient (talking about his follow-up meeting with his former psychologist): I don't think he bothered about what I was saying at all. He doesn't really care about me. I had to repeat myself and he still didn't say anything (possible non-mentalized statement).

Therapist: I can see how you get to that but it also sounds as if he was preoccupied by something else which might explain your impression (offers alternative perspective based on earlier discussion).

Patient: How would I know? He was seeing me and so was supposed to be listening to me whatever else he was doing (explains how he has come to his conclusion).

Therapist: That's right, and it obviously made you feel not wanted, but how did that compare with your feelings for him before (affectively based intervention and suggests further exploration)?

Patient: I used to think that he always listened to me and was interested in what was going on in my life but this . . . . .I won't be going again.

Therapist: It is really upsetting, isn't it, when someone doesn't seem to be how they usually are, but I still wonder if it was because he was preoccupied about something and it has less to do with you as a person. Maybe you were more influenced by that awful feeling of disappointment (links finality of decision to stop seeing her psychologist with problematic feeling that was evoked)?

Patient: Maybe, but when I was there it felt like hard work. But you are right, that was not how he usually was. But it was hurtful.

Therapist: Hmm.

The doing therapist

Early in therapy patients may be unable to imagine that their therapist has them in mind unless special acts of recognition of their needs provide them with explicit and constant evidence that this is the case. Acts are necessary because the teleological character of BPD (see p 23) means that being kept in mind has to be manifest in physical reality. Therapists should expect, at times, to have to demonstrate their understanding through appropriate action within the boundaries of therapy—a supportive letter for housing may be necessary, a telephone call to the patient to help him explore the precipitants of an interpersonal crisis and to monitor what is happening in his mind, or even a home visit with a colleague between sessions in an emergency. Many of these acts can become integral to therapy. A letter written on the patient's behalf should be shared with him before it is sent off and rewritten if necessary as part of the joint attention given to the patient's needs. The first draft by the therapist gives his perspective whilst modification in discussion with the patient demonstrates a process of change and the influence of a mind on a mind. If joint agreement cannot be reached about an aspect of the letter, the therapist must decide whether to remove or retain the opinion. Whichever course of action is taken, the reasons for the decision should be explained to the patient.

The aim of these supportive actions is to develop the therapeutic alliance and to maintain mentalizing by doing it 'out there' in the physical world, showing the patient that you have them in mind. It is not to take over responsibility from the patient. Any actions taken on behalf of the patient should be carefully considered preferably with another team member before they are undertaken and certainly discussed with the team if they have already taken place within a session. This protects against inappropriate enactments.

The monitoring therapist

Being human, you will inevitably make therapy errors, some more serious than others. Here we are not talking about structural mistakes, for example forgetting sessions or failing to organize appointments with due care, but about making interventions that become anti-mentalizing. Gross structural errors require apology, acceptance on your part for your failure and, later, demonstration within the therapy process that you are aware of the effects of the event on your patient.

The mentalizing stance requires you to own up to your own anti-mentalizing errors. You must not to attempt to cover them up or to deny them when confronted. Mistakes are treated as opportunities to revisit what happened and to learn more about contexts, feelings and experiences—'How was it that I did

Box 7.4 **Questions suggesting reflection**

- Is there something I have said or done that might have made you feel like that?
- I am not sure what made me say that. I will have to think about it.
- I believe that I was wrong. What I can't understand is how I came to say it. Can you help me go back to what was happening here before things went wrong?
- Have I missed something that is obvious?

that at that time?' (see Box 7.4). It is not enough to recognize within your own mind that you have made a mistake; alter your behaviour and change your interventions accordingly. You need to articulate what has happened if you are not only to model honesty and courage but above all to demonstrate that you are continually reflecting on what goes on in your mind and on what you do in relation to the patient which is a central component of mentalizing itself.

The irritable therapist and the uncomfortable patient

The hospital out-patient waiting room was placed in a corridor at the entrance to the psychiatric department because of lack of space. A therapist had begun to feel irritated with a new patient because of his focus on complaints about the hospital arrangement, particularly because it seemed to be to the detriment of further discussion about his problems. Although this was only the second session he took his feeling of irritability as countertransference:

Therapist: You seem to feel quite irritable about it today.

Patient: Not really. I think that the way they have organized the clinic doesn't help patients feel relaxed before sessions.

Therapist: So it irritates you that no one does anything about it?

Patient: As I said, I am not particularly irritated by it. I can't understand why they arrange things so patients have to sit in a public area and are seen by everyone who walks past.

Therapist: Maybe you feel a bit irritated with me that I don't do anything about it and have exposed you.

Patient: Will you stop telling me I am irritated? That will make me irritated. Are you sure that's not yours rather than mine?

At this point the therapist is being asked a direct question about his own irritability and has been put on the spot. Perhaps the patient himself is picking something up in the mind of the therapist. What is the therapist to do?

He could continue his line but he has been challenged to reflect about his own state of mind.

> **Therapist:** You know, I think that you are right. I was thinking you were irritated by it, but I realize that it has always irritated me. I was also beginning to consider if your feelings of being looked at in the waiting room though also made it difficult for you to sit here and be looked at by me?

In this situation the therapist has steered a course between accepting his own part in the process and explicitly stated his own contribution. Possibly somewhat bravely he has then linked the situation to the possible current state of mind of the patient in the treatment (interpretative mentalizing).

Countertransference

In contrast to this example mistakes are often a part of countertransference enactment and perhaps using the term 'mistake' is a misnomer. Enactments are inevitable and over-determined, thereby having multiple causes, and should be an expected concomitant of a therapeutic alliance in which the therapist is an essential vehicle for the alien part of the patient's self (see p 15). The mentalizing therapist is not neutral but engaged in a process of reflective enactment (see Box 7.5), making it essential to monitor countertransference because his role is potentially iatrogenic in terms of the interpersonal process. The question for the therapist is what aspect of him contributed to the enactment and what element of the patient stimulated that involvement or what aspect of him provoked the enactment and what did it stimulate in the patient. His reflection about these processes needs to be open and genuinely thoughtful rather than closed and introspective.

Box 7.5 **Reflective enactment**

- Therapist's occasional enactment is acceptable concomitant of therapeutic alliance
- Own up to enactment to rewind and explore
- Check out understanding
- Joint responsibility to understand over-determined enactments
- Monitor your own mistakes
- Model honesty and courage via acknowledgement of your own mistakes—past, current, and future
- Suggest that mistakes offer opportunities to re-visit and learn more about contexts, experiences, and feelings

This sort of joint exploration of possible countertransference experience requires an open-minded therapist, safe in his own failings and appropriately doubtful about his viewpoints so that the patient can manage to open his own mind and begin to question his own rigidly operating schemas about himself and others in the same way that the therapist does. A detached, aloof, refined, defended therapist is unlikely to form a relationship with a patient which helps the patient find himself in the mind of the therapist in an accessible and meaningful way. Borderline patients with their enfeebled capacity for understanding the subjective mental states of others cannot fathom the inscrutability of a remote mind (this therapist stance is most likely to stimulate uncontrolled paranoid reactions). But equally they cannot tolerate one that bubbles with emotion, fails to differentiate different perspectives and exposes them to excessive feelings within the therapist. The therapist needs to become what the patient needs him to be, to feel what the patient wants him to feel but at the same time be able to preserve a part of his mind that mirrors accurately the patient's internal state even following successful projective identification.

It is important to emphasize that this 'mentalizing the countertransference' is not a process of reversal in which the patient is giving the therapist some therapy or the therapist is exploring his own pathology in front of the patient or engaging in self-disclosure (see p 165), all of which are likely to burden the patient rather than help him understand himself. Reflection on enactments or 'mistakes' are by necessity focused on the patient–therapist relationship with both parties being considered as responsible for looking at all the elements that potentially have contributed to the 'error'. This might include the patient's provocative goading and projective processes, on the one hand, or the therapist's sensitivities and unresolved conflicts on the other. This can only be discovered by understanding the mental processes contributing to the error and so a stop, rewind, and explore (see p 133) is necessary, taking the session back before moving it forward again 'frame by frame' or 'mental state by mental state'. Just as behaviours of the patient cannot be understood in isolation from the mental processes that have led to them, so enactments on the part of the therapist cannot become meaningful unless their contributing determinants are identified.

The process therapist

Finally it is important that the therapist concentrates on developing a mentalizing therapeutic process (see Box 7.6) and more attention needs to be devoted to this than to detailed understanding of content. An implicit mentalizing process is a major goal of treatment and this will only develop if the

Box 7.6 **Mentalizing process**

Not directly concerned with content but with helping the patient

+ to generate multiple perspectives →
+ to free themselves up from being stuck in the 'reality' of one view (primary representations and psychic equivalence) →
+ to experience an array of mental states (secondary representations) and →
+ to recognize them as such (meta-representation)

patient can be freed from rigid views held firmly within a schematic belief system. To achieve this shift the therapist should focus on the relationship between patient and therapist as it exemplifies different perspectives and offers opportunities for alternative understanding.

Overt schematic delineation of beliefs will generate explicit mentalization and this forms the basis of many cognitive interventions for BPD. This in itself may be helpful but your goal is the development of an implicit mentalizing process within the therapeutic relationship. Explication of affective states (Box 7.7) embedded within the current transference relationship is therefore emphasized more than cognitive exposition in order to generate an experience of 'feeling felt' in which the patient feels affirmed, validated and not alone and remains in the feeling whilst being aware of the feeling. Our emphasis on process is in line with other dynamic therapies for BPD and those therapists trained in the Conversational Model or Cognitive Analytic Therapy will have little difficulty in recognizing the importance of 'listening' to the process rather than paying too much attention to the exact content (e.g. Meares and Hobson, 1977; Meares, 2000; Ryle, 2004).

One aspect of process that needs special attention is the negotiation of a negative therapeutic reaction or sudden rupture in the alliance which may leave the therapist perplexed and uncertain about how to react. Ruptures frequently result from the conjunction of relationship patterns in patient and therapist (Aveline, 2005), thereby being the product of both rather than one alone; therapists must be skilled in repairing them (Meares, 2000). In our experience the explicitly reflective therapist, who retrieves his own mentalizing ability quickly, following a collapse in the relationship, is the most likely to negotiate severe ruptures in the alliance successfully, and this capacity may be a key factor in maintaining borderline patients in treatment.

Box 7.7 Affective focus and its representation in patient/therapist relationship

- ◆ Focus the patient's attention on therapist experience when it offers an opportunity to clarify misunderstandings and to develop prototypical representations
  - Highlight patient's experience of therapist
  - Use transference to emphasize different experience and perspective
  - Negotiate negative reactions and ruptures in therapeutic alliance by identifying patient and therapist roles in the problem
- ◆ Explication of feelings draws attention back to implicit representations
  - Use language to bolster engagement on the implicit level of mentalization
  - Highlight the experience of 'feeling felt' (mentalized affectivity)

Ruptures represent a failure of mentalizing. The therapist's initial response should be open consideration of his part in the rupture—'what have I said or what is it you feel I have done to bring about this sudden change?'—as a demonstration of a continuing process of self-reflection. This allows the therapist to tease out the different contributions to events in therapy without apportioning blame and firmly embeds the dialogue within the immediacy of the patient–therapist relationship. The gravest danger at these times is increasing your use of those techniques you believe are crucial to patient change and understanding, for example transference interpretation, behavioural challenge and delineation of cognitive distortions. First the therapeutic alliance must be repaired by staying in the rupture and seeking a vantage point from which to view it. You and the patient need to move to a position betwixt and between the heat of the rupture. You both become detectives trying to seek clues about what has happened and this is best done by 'stopping and rewinding' (see p 133) and moving forward to the point of rupture.

In conclusion the therapist stance is inquisitive, active, empathic and at times challenging but most importantly the therapist should refrain from becoming an expert who knows. His mind is focused on the mind of the patient and he is intrigued, questioning and not all-knowing. His primary aim is to stimulate a robust mentalizing process.

Chapter 8

Principles of interventions

In this chapter we discuss some general characteristics of mentalizing interventions and the principles to follow when deciding on the right intervention. As we shall see, being a good therapist is not simply a matter of giving the right intervention. Just as musicians may play most of the right notes but phrase them with inadequate sensitivity, thereby missing the meaning of the piece, so it is only too easy for therapists to make most of the right interventions in therapy but to use them at the wrong moments and without compassion and humanity, rendering therapy hollow. In an attempt to overcome this problem we provide some guiding principles, the first of which is 'if in doubt go back to basics and return to the beginning of our pathway for interventions'. This will help you re-orientate yourself; it is easier to get back on track from a known position. Rather than flailing around in the dark or rushing headlong into danger, if in a hole, stop digging and return to the point at which you felt you knew where both your own and the patient's mind was. In other words whenever you are in considerable doubt and your uncertainty is increasing, return to the basic principles and couple this with a stop, rewind (to a point at which the dialogue was understandable), and explore (see p 133) before moving forward again. There will be many times when the principles are, and should be, broken; being intuitive is an important part of therapy. Here, we can only offer advice that we hope experienced therapists will not find patronizing and condescending. Our training programme is aimed at generic mental health professionals who gallantly implement our treatment without having had extensive therapy training but having had good general experience of risk management, emergency assessment and crisis intervention. Ironically this initial therapeutic naivety of practitioners might be an important part of successful treatment, enabling them to follow basic principles without too much deviation. Experienced therapists have, often necessarily, come to believe in their therapy, their methods and their techniques, and may be in danger of becoming inflexible. Enthusiasts who are setting out on their therapeutic journey and have fewer pre-conceived ideas and hobbyhorses to ride may stand a better chance of taking a mentalizing or 'not-knowing' stance (see p 93). But enough said before we are accused of forming straw-men, stereotypes and archetypes, all of which are examples of non-mentalizing phenomena!

General characteristics of interventions

Interventions should be simple and short rather than long and complex, affect focused rather than concerned with behaviour, target the patient's subjective state of mind rather than a specific aspect of mental activity such as cognition, relate to present events or current interpersonal interactions, be within current mental reality, emphasize near-conscious or conscious content rather than unconscious concerns and be concerned with maintaining process rather than interpreting content.

In general the therapist should avoid inadvertently creating situations where the patient is forced into talking of mental states that they cannot immediately link to subjectively felt reality. A number of simple but hard to observe implications follow from this general rule. First, the therapist who focuses on deep unconscious concerns creates an opportunity for pseudo-mentalization. It is far less risky to stick to conscious or near-conscious content if the therapist's aim is the enhancement of mentalization rather than engendering insight. The former in many ways is commensurate with the latter. It has been argued that therapeutic progress in all therapies is based on achieving representational coherence and integration. Our point here is that while this is arguably best achieved by enhancing insight in less severely disturbed patients, at the more severe end of the spectrum of interpersonal functioning the challenge of a complex mentalizing account somewhat removed from what is consciously accessible can generate disintegration and incoherence of the representational world. This is a simple point but an all-important one. If a person is struggling with maintaining a grip over the massive distortions of their subjective experience, an expert who describes complex mental states of conflict, ambivalence

---

Box 8.1 General characteristics of interventions

- Simple and short
- Affect focused (love, desire, hurt, catastrophe, excitement)
- Focus on patient's mind (not on behaviour)
- Relate to current event or activity—mental reality (evidence based or in working memory)
- De-emphasize unconscious concerns in favour of near-conscious or conscious content

and non-conscious motives is more likely to generate turmoil than bring about integration. Probably turmoil of that sort is created in patients with less severe disturbance as well when the complexity of their mental functioning is brought to the foreground of consciousness. However, against a background of competence in dealing with subjective experience such turmoil can be the catalyst for reorganization. In borderline patients sensitized to the possibility of confusion it undermines rather than enhances a fledgling capacity for finding real meaning behind behaviour. Thus you should be less concerned with use of metaphor, analogies, puns and symbolism. These latter aspects of interventions require a high level of mentalizing and are likely only to be beneficial in furthering understanding at those moments when the borderline patient is able to balance internal emotional states with inner reflection. At other times such interventions will be met either with incomprehension, envious admiration, dismissal or development of pretend mode (see p 73).

The clever therapist

A patient complained that her housing association had done nothing about the leak in the roof of her flat. She had reported it a number of times but workmen had still not visited to repair the roof. She believed that her flat would flood if it rained too hard and her furniture would be ruined.

Therapist: Perhaps you feel that I am doing nothing to repair the leak that has opened up in your mind, and if I don't do something quickly your feelings will get out of control and ruin everything?

Patient: They should come round and repair it. I got angry with them again and soon I will go around and 'start' on them if they don't come.

Therapist: So then your feelings really are going to leak badly at that point?

Patient: Stop going on about my feelings, will you. You would be frustrated if people didn't turn up to repair things, wouldn't you. So stop making out that what I am feeling is a problem. It is only a problem because they haven't done what they are supposed to do.

The session continued in this way until the therapist stopped trying to link the practical problem to what was happening in the therapy. It is not so much that the therapist is wrong here but that the timing is off-beat and the patient cannot increase her self-reflection when trapped in her mind about a very practical issue. Her current mental reality is fixed within a teleological mode at this point and so drawing analogous links is relatively meaningless to her.

Simple and short

Keeping things simple and short is easier said than done, but the principle is to ensure that your interventions are in keeping with the patient's mentalizing capacity. The longer and more complex interventions become, the less likely they are to be within the patient's mentalizing ability, particularly if he is emotionally aroused at the time. The mentalizing capacity of borderline patients fluctuates according to the attachment system's level of stimulation. Thus, at one moment a patient may be able to understand and react to a complex intervention and yet at another unable to comprehend or even listen to something straightforward. The more you stimulate the emotional state of the patient and increase the arousal of the attachment system the more fragile their mentalizing capacity becomes and so the therapist must tread more carefully in their interventions.

Affect focused

All dynamic therapies are concerned with emotional states. In MBT affect focused means grasping the affect in the immediacy of the moment, not so much in its relation to the content of the session but primarily as it relates to what is currently happening between patient and therapist. A brief intervention identifying the current feeling between patient and therapist is likely to propel a session forward more effectively than focusing on the detail of the content of a narrative.

Sexual encounters

A patient told her therapist about the frequent brief sexual encounters she had. As she was telling her about them and how she met her partners on night buses she moved from a position of defiant justification to wary uncertainty.

Therapist: Just then you seemed to be less sure (grasping the immediate affect shift).

Patient: I don't care what people think. I do it because I like it and I have fun anyway.

Therapist: You sound a little defiant, maybe against me?

Silence

Therapist: It seemed for a moment that you did care what I thought or something came into your mind about it. Perhaps you felt I might enjoy listening to your conquests or the opposite that I might disapprove.

Patient: My friends always ask about them and they don't disapprove.

Therapist: But I am not your friend.

Patient: You can say that again! What do you think about my exploits? Are you a bit of a prude?

Therapist: Not many people think I am a prude! It is not for me to be moralistic about what you do. What I do think is that it sounds as if you are putting yourself at risk and that is a problem for us because we are working on your risky behaviour, but it sounds like you don't feel it is a problem for you at the moment.

Patient: I didn't say that. There have been times when it has all gone wrong and something unpleasant has happened. One of them beat me up.

In this vignette the therapist focuses on the immediate change in affect during the dialogue and at the same time begins to introduce an alternative perspective to the patient's attitude to her risky behaviour.

Focus on the patient's mind not on behaviour

In working with challenging patients who have the propensity to act rather than think, to behave rather than feel, the temptation is always to engage with them at the level at which they are expressing themselves. This means first of all that the therapist is always tempted to respond by action. The patient challenges by self-harm or direct aggression, is irritable and uncommunicative. The therapist feels obliged to react to this behaviour, in the first instance perhaps by providing excessively complex explanations and in the face of a lack of response increasingly to act themselves. We must remember that talking is action and a verbal response may be a behavioural reaction to the patient's apparent bloody-mindedness. A therapist's excessive verbalization following a piece of challenging behaviour from the patient may be experienced by the patient as 'punishment', in part because it is, whatever the conscious intention might have been.

The telling indicator is the therapist's focus on the patient's behaviour rather than the patient's mind. The therapist often reacts to a piece of enactment by forcing the patient to talk about it, at times rubbing the patient's nose into the 'mess' they have created by forcing the patient to find meaning behind their action. An innocent question such as, 'We need to understand why you felt you needed to cut yourself today' is not likely to enhance the patient's capacity to mentalize. Rather, it forces them to focus on the behaviour they engaged in that itself was a consequence of a failure of mentalization. The mentalizing therapist knows that this is precisely what the patient is incapable of doing: finding and giving a reason for their action. If they could, they might not have needed to do it. Forcing them to face up to their actions is a non-mentalizing and unnecessarily confrontative shaming and undermining act that at best calls forth pseudo-mentalization.

The therapist needs to be able to set aside the behaviour, not in the sense of pretending it didn't happen but in the sense of playing Sherlock Holmes in relation to it and get on with her/his task of focusing on the patient's mind. A starting point for such a focus may be the impact that the behaviour had on the patient himself. Something like, 'You know, it wouldn't surprise me if you felt disappointed with yourself after you did this because you were trying so hard to stop doing it'. Perhaps later on the focus can shift to the patient's state of mind that precedes the challenging behaviour in question. Of course this implies causation, but this does not mean asking the patient to make a link between their actions and the mental state antecedents. The therapist uses the action as an indicator that a feeling or a thought must have arisen in a relational context which created a high level of arousal, intensified the activation of the attachment system or reinforced a tendency towards phobic avoidance and caused a general collapse of mentalization. The therapist thus focuses on the patient's mind as it struggles with experiences before the behaviour in question. For example, an act of aggression may have followed a relatively neutral discussion with the patient concerning their plans after the treatment ended. The therapist observes that the patient becomes increasingly agitated, and after the end of the conversation the patient attacks the furniture and breaks a potted plant. The therapist's task is to reach back and see what it was about the conversation that might have caused the collapse of mentalization. In this case, the patient's anxiety about the future and their sense of helplessness, which is mismatched by the therapist's expectation of the patient's ability to cope, may well have caused the collapse of thinking. The therapist addresses the issue by apologizing and acknowledging that unintentionally she placed a massive burden on the patient by talking as if she assumed the patient would definitely be able to cope while the patient felt quite uncertain about their own capacity.

Relate to current event or activity

Often when working psychotherapeutically we seek refuge in the past. Although the current trend within psychotherapies is for so-called here and now interpretative work, this is generally recognized as more anxiety provoking than reaching into the past, working with memories of childhood experience, forging causal links between current behaviour and past events and the subjective experiences these *might have generated*. Explaining a person's current wish to please in terms of a continuing wish to satisfy a demanding image of a parent may be an easier way of tackling an interpersonal problem than looking at the patient's overarching desire to please the therapist and thereby sabotage genuine interaction. Reaching into the past can be more comfortable but also far less real and thus encourage pseudo-mentalizing about what the patient might or might not have felt as a child or the parents might or might not have thought all those years ago.

The best way of circumventing this potential difficulty is by selectively focusing on recent experiences outside of the therapeutic situation or the situation in the room at the moment. This is not quite the same as the psychoanalytic focus often characterized ironically as 'you mean me' interpretations. That kind of work can also lead to pseudo-mentalizing in borderline patients. The general principle concerns a preference for focusing on emotionally charged but perhaps relatively trivial events around which the thoughts and feelings of the protagonists may be productively elaborated.

In general the therapist aims to work with whatever is current in the patient's mind; in other words, in working memory. It is important that the experience should have mental reality for the patient, that it should feel like a real experience when talked about. Thus at times experiences long ago can have this kind of sense of currency. The therapist must be careful, however, that the mental reality associated with it has 'real depth' rather than a stereotypic repetitive reproduction, a kind of mantra where it is the experience of recall that is real rather than the reality of the experience.

Clinical pathway for interventions

In principle, the pathway for interventions progresses from dealing with: (1) affects in relation to current external interpersonal relationships; (2) to affects in relation to themes within treatment (e.g. how the patient interacts within the programme); and (3) finally to affects, immediate aspects of the patient–therapist relationship and the intrapsychic state of the patient (see Box 8.2).

The overall aim in moving along the pathway is to stimulate a natural therapeutic process that becomes almost expected with the emphasis being less on content and more on process as both therapist and patient move around the anchor points flexibly. This order of movement between interventions is a principle and not a rule and there will be many times when it is necessary to jump levels and mix levels. Following the pathway will move the patient from

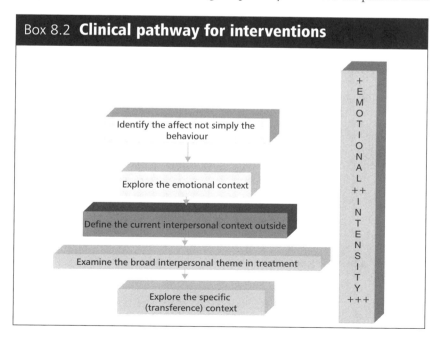

Box 8.2 **Clinical pathway for interventions**

Identify the affect not simply the behaviour

Explore the emotional context

Define the current interpersonal context outside

Examine the broad interpersonal theme in treatment

Explore the specific (transference) context

+ EMOTIONAL ++ INTENSITY +++

the least intensely felt introspection to the most intensely felt as long as the therapist remains focused on affects and the interpersonal domain. Clearly there are exceptions to this generalization and at times, focusing on the emotional interaction between patient and therapist, usually the most concentrated emotional area, may be rendered cold and intellectual and represent a move away from the heat of an external or treatment context—an example of playing the right notes but without regard for appropriate phrasing.

Taking each step in turn, the therapist starts from identifying affects and does not focus solely on behaviour. This requires the therapist to ask questions such as 'What were you feeling at that point?' rather than asking 'What did you do next?'; 'What are you feeling now?' rather than 'What do you think you should do?'. This is a false dichotomy of course, but the emphasis of the dialogue should be on the affect and not the behaviour even when exploring suicidal and self-destructive behaviour (see p 113).

Having identified affects, the emotional and/or interpersonal context external to the therapy session related to the feelings should be explored. This will happen quite naturally as you attempt to define underlying emotions. Appraisal of outside interpersonal interactions is immediately meaningful to borderline patients and, when discussed 'after the event', is less likely to induce the powerful emotions evoked at the time of the interaction. So, making time for retrospective reflection allows the patient and therapist to 'strike whilst the iron is cold' or better still 'whilst it is cooling down'—mentalizing interpersonal events without too much danger of mental collapse or loss of attention. Similar work can be done within an individual therapy session about a patient's interactions within an earlier group session, for example, reflecting on what *was* rather than what *is*. Whilst this is no substitute for a patient addressing his feelings in the heat of the moment, in our experience, the ability to reflect and to act constructively whilst emotionally aroused gradually develops only as the person is able to consider his and others' states of mind retrospectively. We all reflect with greater honesty with hindsight than we do within the hurly burly of an emotional interaction itself, but in the end our lives are led and possibly determined within the subjective immediacy of interactions, and borderline patients need to learn to use these moments constructively.

We are not recommending downgrading therapeutic work within the immediacy of the patient-therapist relationship; in fact we recommend quite the opposite. However, it is important to move towards working in this way with sensitivity, without overwhelming the patient with emotional states that he cannot understand or address. Moving too quickly and without adequate preparation will stimulate a gradual failure in mentalizing, which if uncontrolled may lead to a crisis in the session and become iatrogenic (see Chapter 3), provoking the very behaviours you seek to address.

Which intervention when?

We have defined a number of interventions in keeping with dynamic and other therapies. These are discussed in more detail in Chapter 9. Here we identify the principles to follow in deciding which intervention to use at any given moment. We have arranged the interventions in order of complexity, depth and emotional intensity, with empathy and support being the simplest most superficial and least intensive, and mentalizing the transference being the most complex and, for the most part, the most emotionally intensive. Commonly, the decision about which intervention to use when will be taken outside consciousness and be all the better for it but we believe that there are some general principles to follow. These are summarized in Box 8.4.

Box 8.3 Spectrum of interventions

- Reassurance, support, and empathy
- Clarification, challenge, and elaboration
- Basic mentalizing
- Interpretive mentalizing
- Mentalizing the transference
- Non-mentalizing interpretations—use with care

Box 8.4 Which intervention to use when?

- If in doubt start at the surface—support and empathy
- Move to 'deeper' levels only after you have performed the earlier steps
- If emotions are in danger of becoming overwhelming take a step towards the surface
- Type of intervention is inversely related to emotional intensity—support and empathy being given when the patient is overwhelmed with emotion; mentalizing transference when the patient can continue mentalizing whilst 'holding' the emotion.
- Intervention must be in keeping with the patient's mentalizing capacity at the time at which it is given. The danger is in assuming that border-line patients have a greater capacity than they actually have when they are struggling with feelings.

The basis for our recommendations is simply that, in general, mentalizing capacity in borderline patients is inversely related to stimulation of the attachment system. As the attachment system is activated the capacity to mentalize is inhibited; emotions become bewildering, the self fractures and actions to restore precarious safety and sense of balance become inevitable. This process causes the well-described volatile pattern of relationships of intimacy and distance, found in patients with BPD who try to maintain their mind when it becomes overwhelmed. It is senseless to reproduce this pattern in an uncontrolled manner early in therapy by over-stimulating the patient, inducing complex mental states and provoking highly evocative emotions. Balancing stimulation of the attachment system with capacity to mentalize places the therapist in the delicate position of having to mobilize affect whilst controlling its flow and intensity. Without emotion there can be no meaningful subjective experience but with excess emotion there can be no understanding of the subjective experience.

As we have argued before, one of the gravest dangers for therapists treating borderline patients is iatrogenic harm by using well-meaning but mistimed and misguided interventions that diminish rather than increase mentalizing capacity through excessive activation of the attachment system. Therefore the overarching principle to be followed when selecting interventions is to minimize iatrogenic effects by balancing emotional intensity with the patient's continuing capacity to subjectively monitor his own mind and that of another.

At the surface level, sensitively given support and empathy are unlikely to provoke complex mental states in borderline patients who, feeling someone else is showing interest and is attempting to understand their emotional state from their point of view, will feel safe enough to explain their feelings and give their perspective about what has happened or is happening to them. The patient's mind is not threatened. Hence these types of interventions, along with motivational interviewing, problem solving, psychoeducation and other behavioural techniques, are useful early in therapy.

At the intermediate level of intervention, challenge creates more difficulty because it forces self-scrutiny and implies another mind might have a different perspective that has to be considered and integrated. If the challenge incorporates interpersonal content and current affect rather than being intellectual it forms part of basic mentalizing because the relational world is invoked which heightens the emotional intensity. If the intervention is then linked to 'you and me' and underlying motivations are brought into play the danger of overwhelming the patient's mentalizing capacity increases considerably, as does that of inducing action. The patient walks out of a session or cuts himself to restore his mind. This cascade of psychological disaster can be avoided if therapists move slowly down the levels of intervention, only reaching the greatest depth having worked on the earlier levels first. You should only move down a level when you judge the patient's degree of anxiety, and therefore mentalizing capacity allows him to consider your perspective further or he himself is willing to elaborate more. If in doubt your interventions should be tentative at first and you should only inject more pressure into the dialogue when the therapeutic relationship is robust.

It is not our intention to suggest that therapists must adhere rigidly to the principles outlined here. But if therapists follow our clinical pathway and sensibly implement our recommendations about timing of interventions we believe they will be less at risk of causing harm and will have the greatest chance of stimulating a positive therapeutic relationship within which mentalizing can flourish.

Basic principles—a clinical example

We are commonly asked how to deal with many of the critical issues that beset borderline patients and their therapists. It is impossible to outline how to manage every situation and so we urge clinicians to follow the basic principles that we have set out in this chapter. The most difficult behaviours for therapists are suicide attempts and self-harm. Here we outline the principles once again in relation to these behaviours.

Suicide attempts and self-harm

To reiterate some of the principles—interventions should be simple and short, affect focused, refer to the current/immediate context, and initially address conscious or near-conscious content. The pathway for interventions moves from affect identification to interpersonal context to meaning and therefore moves from surface to depth only when the emotional state allows reflective mentalizing. Finally, it is important to adopt a non-judgemental attitude to suicide attempts and self-harm or other destructive activities and to refrain from assuming that it is an action aimed at the treatment itself or even to attack you (see Box 8.5).

The therapist should not assume responsibility for the patient's actions and a comment early in treatment defining the extent of his responsibility is necessary, for example:

> I can't stop you harming yourself or even killing yourself, but I might be able to help you understand what makes you try to do it and to find other ways of managing things.

The primary purpose of self-harm and other actions is to maintain self-structure following sudden destabilization. It is not to express aggression or to

---

Box 8.5 **Function of self-harm**

- To maintain the self-structure
  - Explore reasons for destabilization of self-structure
    - 'Tell me when you first began to feel anxious that you might do something?'
  - Make a systematic attempt to place responsibility for actions back with the patient to re-establish self-control
    - 'I can't stop you harming yourself or even killing yourself but I might be able to help you understand what makes you do it and to find other ways of managing things.'

Box 8.6 **Motivation of self-harm**

- Re-stabilize
  - Predictable, mentalizable schematic relationships
  - Rigid understandable motivations—'He didn't turn up because he wanted me to suffer'.
  - Formulaic explanations—'He deserves to suffer because he is bad'. 'I won't come because they don't want me there'.
- Reduce panic
- Establish existence
  - Support for body existence through seeing blood
  - When mental existence is in doubt reinforce existence through your body
  - Emptiness becomes partially filled
- Rarely to control/attack other

---

attack someone else. Whilst the motivations are complex (see Box 8.6) we suggest that self-harm and suicide attempts occur when mental existence is in doubt and personal integrity can only be re-established through the body with blood, for example, supporting existence within the teleological understanding of the patient at that moment. Emptiness and absence become partially filled by the action.

Intervention

Start at the beginning of the pathway using supportive and empathic interventions and establish the events of the self-harm including any interpersonal context.

'You mustn't have known what else to do'; 'It must be disappointing to you after all this time when you have worked so hard not to do it'.

In defining the interpersonal context (see box 8.7 and box 8.8), gently explore who the patient was with or who he was thinking about before it happened. Find out when the feelings leading to self-harm began by taking the patient back to a point when he was clear that he did not feel like harming himself in any compulsive way—a rewind and explore (see p 133) (many patients treasure self-harm in the back of their mind as a way of managing feeling states but this is not the same as the compulsive urge that builds up as the solution pushes forward which is what the therapist is trying to identify here). The emphasis needs to be on feeling states as part of an overall mental state and not on cognitive states or antecedent triggers and so the dialogue is more about how the context interacts with the feelings and mental state of the patient— 'What was going on in your mind at the time?' In particular, look out for communication difficulties and oversensitivity which lead to difficulties in managing feelings of rejection, abandonment, humiliation or conversely powerful feelings of love, desire and need that lead to destabilization of the self and a flood of affect overwhelming the mind. Remember that within the

---

Box 8.7 Pathway and interventions for self-harm

- Empathy and support
- Define interpersonal context
  - Detailed account of days or hours leading up to self-harm with emphasis on feeling states
  - Moment to moment exploration of actual episode
  - Explore communication problems
  - Identify misunderstandings or over-sensitivity
- Identify affect
  - Explore the affective changes since the previous individual session linking them with events within treatment
  - Review any acts thoroughly in a number of contexts including individual and group therapy

Box 8.8 **Interventions for self-harm**

DO

- Explore conscious motive
  - How do you understand what happened?
  - Who was there at the time or who were you thinking about?
  - What did you make of what they said?
- Challenge the perspective that the patient presents

DO NOT

- Mentalize the transference in the immediacy of a suicide attempt or self-harm
- Interpret the patient's actions in terms of their personal history, the putative unconscious motivations or their current possible manipulative intent in the 'heat' of the moment. It will alienate the patient.

context of a collapse of the mind borderline patients experience feelings at the level of psychic equivalence. Thus 'feeling bad' becomes 'I am bad'. Your interventions must reflect a sense that you understand this and are not underestimating the power of their experience.

Initially the conscious determinants of the self-harm should be explored without trying to second guess more complex psychological reasons. But within this exploration the patient's explanation should be questioned if it is schematic and formulaic, because these are non-mentalizing phenomena and will prevent the development of an appropriate mental buffer to future experiences which might lead to self-harm. The patient's actions should not be interpreted in terms of their personal history, the putative unconscious motivations or their current possible manipulative intent in the 'heat' of the moment. This will alienate the patient. Only later will you be able to build up evidence for underlying unconscious determinants and then you can 'strike whilst the iron is cold' or 'cooling down' in relation to the self-harm but 'hot' in relation to the transference interaction. It may be possible to do this within one session but more often it needs to be done over a few sessions.

Illustrative clinical example

The abandoned cutter

A patient talked about her self-laceration the previous day, glossing over what had happened and insisting that it was unimportant.

Therapist: Tell me a bit more about what happened?

Patient: There is nothing more to say really. I cut myself with the cup I broke when I threw it against the wall after I got home.

Therapist: Let's go back and tell me when you first began to feel something was wrong. (A rewind of the content.)

Patient: I don't know really.

Therapist: Bear with me; can you remember what you felt yesterday for example in the group? (Trying to identity a therapy context.)

Patient: No. I was OK after that and I think I was when I got home early in the evening. I arranged to see two of my friends as I said and it was only when I got home after that I began to feel miserable.

Therapist: So you were aware that you were miserable at that point. It sounds like something might have occurred during the evening.

The session continued in this way with the therapist insisting on exploring the detail of the miserable affect. It turned out that the patient had felt abandoned (an earlier feeling to the misery) by her two friends when they had gone off to the toilet together and left her alone for what she felt was an excessive length of time.

Patient: I felt so hurt (a further affect complicating the internal state of the patient at that time) that I nearly cut myself then with my knife but I scratched myself with my finger nails to get a bit of blood out instead. Then I got the idea that I should just get up and go so that when they came back they would not know where I was (motive of revenge appears to have been stimulated by the severe scratching; only with a mentalizing mind can the patient have revenge feelings which require self and other and hence her revenge fantasy occurs after she has scratched herself) but just as I was about to go they came back.

Therapist: And?

Patient: I didn't say anything at all. What's the point? They had already spent ages and that couldn't be undone.

Therapist: So you felt excluded and a bit angry and didn't know what to do about how you felt. Scratching yourself made you a bit clearer and you momentarily became revengeful before becoming miserable later. I guess that again cutting was the only way you could make things feel better then.

(Therapist is focusing on affective relief from cutting and also hinting at stabilizing effect of the action—it brings back the patient's mind at the point at which it is lost. Cutting and other actions are ways of reinstating a mentalizing mind.)

Patient: It always clears how I feel and then I can get on with things again. I was able to watch TV for a time and then go to bed without dwelling on it all.

Therapist: But you cut yourself again.

Patient: Soon after I got home I felt awful again and so really wanted to do it that time.

Therapist: It seems that you cut yourself to get rid of feelings that you don't know what to do with and as a way to get your mind back. You could think of taking revenge when you scratched yourself badly but your friends thwarted you by coming back. Maybe afterwards your mind was taken over again by feelings and you could only get things straight in your head when you cut?.

Patient: It made me feel an OK person and somehow helped me know what was me and what was them. It doesn't matter.

Therapist: I think that it does matter because when you feel left out and on your own, your mind starts to disappear and you don't know what is going on and it reminds me of the time when I was late for a session and you cut yourself in the toilet. I think that when you have feelings like that you begin to believe that you are not worth anything and that that is what I was saying about you by being late and what your friends were saying when they went off. Cutting brings you back to some semblance of being someone (interpretive mentalizing and moving towards mentalizing the transference (see p 139)).

Patient: You know that I started cutting when I was 18. I really found it comforting then and I still do. I know that I get confused and I am addicted to it now when I am like that.

Chapter 9

The mentalizing focus and basic interventions

In MBT the therapist's goal is to learn more about how a person is thinking and feeling. This requires the therapist to constantly explore the current state of mind of the patient whilst putting forward his own understanding of the patient's state of mind. The purpose is to stimulate the patient to use his own mind further to understand his mental states and those of others, including the therapist's. The therapist's task is to develop this joint process in therapy and to maintain the mentalizing focus throughout treatment. When the patient questions your view, you should give a clear explanation of how you have come to your opinion and express any uncertainties you have about your perspective. As the interaction develops, you may change your mind about your understanding of the patient's experience and you should be able to demonstrate this to the patient if further mentalizing is to be stimulated. A statement from a therapist such as 'I understand now what you are saying. That means that what I said is not quite right. Perhaps it is more like . . .' is a valuable way to stimulate mentalizing in the patient and to demonstrate interpersonal respect. This 'models' reflectiveness and allows the patient to recognize that having one's mind changed by another mind is not humiliating but constructive and developmental in a relationship.

There are a number of techniques that are likely to promote mentalizing. Many of these are well known to therapists; you may well begin to feel as you read this section that you are already doing much of what is described here. Our aim is not to teach new techniques but to recommend that you focus therapy differently by placing greater emphasis on some aspects of treatment whilst reducing others.

Motivation

Motivation to change and enthusiasm for treatment is highly variable in borderline patients. Small changes, such as holidays, illness, or room changes may have serious consequences for treatment. As a therapist you must be constantly alert to decreases in motivation and alter your interaction with the

> ## Box 9.1 **Maintaining motivation**
>
> - Demonstrate support, reassurance and empathy as you explore the patient's mind
> - Model reflectivity
> - Identify the discrepancy between the experience of the self and the ideal self—'how you are, compared with how you would like to be'
> - 'Go with the flow' or 'roll with the resistance' for a short time
> - Re-appraise gains and identify continuing problem areas
> - Highlight competencies in mentalization and listen for mentalizing strengths

patient accordingly. As a generalization the level of motivation is inversely proportional to the patient's degree of agitation and emotional distress. The patient will not be able to maintain a state of reflective thoughtfulness about treatment when their arousal overwhelms their ability to process feelings and experiences.

A great deal has been written about maintaining motivation and much of it has been part of good therapeutic technique for many years. Even if you have not been trained in the specific techniques there are a number of principles that will help you maintain a patient's motivation for treatment which are in line with a focus on mentalization. These are summarized in Box 9.1.

Reassurance, support, and empathy

Reassurance, support, and empathy are necessary components of all therapies and the therapeutic skills of reflective listening and accurate empathy are a fundamental aspect of MBT. They are not the same as agreeing with everything the patient says and, as we shall see, confrontation or challenge is an equally important aspect of therapy. However, they are synonymous with listening non-judgementally, refraining from criticism and abstaining from guessing about how a patient feels. Open questions are the road to reassurance—'Tell me a bit more about the problem'. As the patient explores in detail how he feels about something, a quiet nod of encouragement from the therapist may be all that is required. Positive and hopeful questioning will also provide some reassurance for the patient and demonstrates your desire to know and to understand the problems. You will have to constantly 'check-out' your understanding—'As I have understood, what you have been saying is . . .' 'Does that sound right'?

Box 9.2 **Supportive attitude**

- Respectful of patient narrative and expression
- Positive/hopeful attitude but questioning
- Unknowing stance—you cannot know their position
- Demonstrate a desire to know and to understand
- Constantly check back your understanding
- Spell out emotional impact of narrative based on common sense psychology and personal experience
- For the patient but not acting for them—retains patient responsibility

---

Inexperienced practitioners confuse having theoretical knowledge and being aware of their own life experience with knowing the answers and may believe that giving advice is in itself supportive. But using your theoretical knowledge without teasing out the patient's perspective is likely to lead to gross assumptions on your part, diminish the individuality of the patient's problems and gradually move the patient-therapist relationship towards one in which the patient passively looks to the therapist for answers and the therapist unwittingly gives suggestions or uses problem-solving techniques excessively. The aim in MBT is not to act for the patient but to remain alongside the patient helping him explore areas of uncertainty and to develop meaning. The therapist needs to keep an image in his mind of two people looking at a map, trying to decide which way to go; although they may have agreed on the final destination, neither party knows the route, and indeed there may be many ways to reach the destination.

Empathic statements are a way to deepen the rapport between patient and therapist but accurately reflecting underlying emotional states may be more problematic in treatment of borderline patients than in others. Borderline patients cannot readily discern their own subjective state and they cannot benefit from being told how they feel. You must refrain from telling the patient what they are saying or what they are 'really feeling'; some examples of proscribed statements in MBT are given in Box 9.3.

The problem is compounded if the therapist persists in telling the patient what his underlying feeling is or what he is really saying and for good measure gives him the underlying reasons as well. This results in one of two possible negative responses. On the one hand, it may lead to passive acquiescence and acceptance that the therapist 'knows' things about the patient that the patient

> ## Box 9.3 **Proscribed statements**
>
> - What you really feel is . . .
> - I think what you are really telling me is . . .
> - It strikes me that what you are really saying . . .
> - I think your expectations of this situation are distorted
> - What you meant is . . .

doesn't know; on the other hand, it may result in inappropriate bickering about who is right. In essence, the therapist stance has moved away from the mentalizing or 'not-knowing' stance to one of superiority and dominance. Such a stance is likely to lead to enactments between patient and therapist and may create problems within the therapy that are a product of the therapy itself rather than specific to the borderline patient.

Identifying and exploring positive mentalizing

Appropriate use of praise creates a reassuring atmosphere within therapy and positive attitudes from the therapist are commonly used to instil hope and to suggest a pathway for change. The question is when to use praise. We do not suggest that the therapist is unwaveringly positive and encouraging but that the therapist expressly recognises when a patient has used mentalizing with positive results (see Box 9.4).

The principle to follow is: use praise judiciously to highlight positive mentalizing and to explore its beneficial effects.

The therapist alights on how the patient has understood a complex interpersonal situation, for example, and examines how this may have helped him not only to understand how he felt but also to recognize the other person's feelings.

> 'My mother phoned me and asked me to come to help her pack before she went on holiday. I told her I wasn't going to do that. She said that I had always been a selfish girl given all that she did for me, which of course upset me. This time though I didn't put the phone down but told her that I couldn't help her pack because I had to go to work. She made me feel guilty about that but I said that it was too late for me to ask for time off. In the end I was able to say that I would also miss her because of all she did for me. The therapist said 'you sound like you really managed to explain something to her this time. How did that make you feel?' Later he explored how the patient thought her mother felt about the whole conversation. The patient and her mother had managed to say goodbye to each other in a constructive way which seemed to leave them both feeling satisfied at the end of the phone call.

Box 9.4 Identifying and exploring positive mentalizing

- Judicious praise—'you have really managed to understand what went on between you'
- Examine how it feels to others when such mentalizing occurs—'how do you think they felt about it when you explained it to them?'
- Explore how it feels to self when an emotional situation is mentalized—'how did working that out make you feel?'
- Identify non-mentalizing fillers, for example, trite explanations
- Highlight fillers and explore lack of practical success associated with them

Box 9.5 Provoking curiosity about motivations

- Highlight own interest in 'why'
- Qualify own understanding and inferences—'I can't be sure but'; 'maybe you'; 'I guess that you'
- Guide patient's focus towards experience and away from 'fillers'
- Demonstrate how such information could help to make sense of things

The therapist should not become a 'cheerleader' supporting the patient from the touchline but stand alongside the patient provoking curiosity about motivations and demonstrating how understanding and explaining to oneself and others improves emotional satisfaction and control of mood states (see Box 9.5).

Judicious praise of mentalizing strengths is balanced by identification of non-mentalizing 'fillers'. Trite explanations, dismissive statements, assumptions, rationalizations, etc., should all be identified and tackled as they arise. Most non-mentalizing fillers do not help to develop relationships and understanding of situations or oneself and this needs to be highlighted.

The use of these non-mentalizing fillers may enable the patient to avoid problems or ensure that current explanations and understanding do not have to be reviewed or changed. The therapist must make sure that the patient recognizes that this is avoidance and defensiveness and seek to bring the patient back to a focus on his current state of mind.

Clarification and affect elaboration

Clarification is self-explanatory and requires little elucidation here. It is the 'tidying up' or making meaning of and giving context to behaviour which has resulted from a failure of mentalization (see Box 9.6).

In order to 'tidy up', important facts have to be established and their relationship to underlying feelings identified. Actions should always be traced to feelings whenever possible by rewinding the events and establishing the moment by moment process leading to an action. Within this process the therapist should be alert to any failures to 'read minds' or to understand one's own mind and when this is apparent in the story he should question it and seek an alternative understanding of the failed mentalization. Open questions, re-stating facts, and focusing on moment-to-moment events are common clarification techniques.

A 22 year old patient reported that he had left his university course. He had failed to attend lectures and seminars for a few weeks, preferring to stay at home and smoke cannabis. The first time he re-attended his tutor asked him where he had been. Taking offence he told him—'stick your course up your . . .' —and then walked out. He had not returned after that. The therapist asked the patient to go back to the point at which he had stopped attending the university lectures and traced events leading up to his absence. Having spent considerable time looking at preceding events and tracing the pathway to the patient's eventual return to university the therapist alighted on the obvious failure of mentalization when the student shouted at his tutor and walked out. In the transcription of the tape the therapist makes many comments such as 'Take me through what happened'; 'Not so quickly. Can you go slowly there and tell me what was in your mind at the time'; 'Just to be clear—you felt that your tutor was criticising you and sneering about your lack of attendance'; 'Looking back do you think that what he said could have been meant any other way?'; 'Have there been other times when you have felt he didn't like you?' These are all attempts to clarify the pathway leading up to the failure of mentalization whilst linking it to what was going

Box 9.6 **Clarification**

- ◆ Tidying up of behaviour which has resulted from a failure of mentalization
- ◆ Establish important 'facts' from patient perspective
- ◆ Reconstruct the events
- ◆ Make behaviour explicit—extensive detail of actions and associated feelings
- ◆ Avoid mentalizing the behaviours at this point
- ◆ Trace action to feeling
- ◆ Seek indicators of lack of reading of minds

on in his mind at the time. It transpired that his understanding of his tutor's mind was that he was being censorious when in fact an alternative understanding was that his tutor was expressing concern for him and showing that he had missed him. In an attempt to link the patient's experience of the motive behind his tutor's question to his action, the therapist asked what the tutor would have had to say and perhaps have thought about for him to have felt differently and not to have acted so precipitously.

Affect elaboration requires the therapist to explore empathically the feeling states of the patient (see Box 9.7) and not to be deflected from the task by manifest feelings.

Many patients will express feelings during the session or talk about how they felt under specific circumstances and in MBT, because there is a particular focus on the affective state of the patient, this is encouraged. But the therapist should keep in mind that the affect focus in MBT is primarily on the predominant feeling in a moment of the session as manifest between patient and therapist—the here-and-now rather than the there-and-then (see p 108).

It is important to elicit feelings during non-mentalizing interactions. Strong affects disrupt mentalizing. As the patient becomes increasingly bewildered about feelings his mental agitation increases, quickly overwhelming his capacity to be reflective. Physical agitation, actions, panic and defensive manoeuvres result. Identifying feelings and placing them in context helps to reduce the perplexity of the patient and reduces the likelihood that feelings have to be managed through self-harm or other actions.

Many patients exhibit emotions that are unlikely to induce sympathy in others. The expression of such feelings should become a focus of therapy if it seems likely that the overtly expressed emotion covers a feeling that is more likely to provoke a caring or concerned response from someone else. A common example of this process is the use of anger and hostility to cover more

---

Box 9.7 Affect elaboration

◆ During non-mentalizing interaction therapist firmly tries to elicit feeling states

◆ Therapist recognizes mixed emotions—probe for other feelings than first, particularly if first emotion is unlikely to provoke sympathy in others or lead to rejection (e.g. frustration, or anger)

◆ Reflect on what it must be like to feel like that in that situation

◆ Try to learn from individual what would need to happen to allow them to feel differently

◆ How would you need others to *think about you*, to feel differently?

problematic feelings such as closeness and intimacy. Here the therapist should make careful use of countertransference feelings that may be the first indication of the patient's underlying state.

Stop and stand—challenge or trip

The therapist has one primary aim when using stop and stand (see Box 9.8)—to reinstate mentalizing when it fails, either in himself or in the patient. This is in itself not a challenge but defines the manoeuvre of the therapist at the moment when mentalizing shifts dramatically. The therapist interrupts the dialogue of the session to insist that the patient focuses on the moment of rupture in order to reinstate mentalizing. If it is his own failure of mentalizing, for example, becoming muddled in a group, the technique is used to re-establish the process within himself. Stop and stand is both a breathing space and a pivotal moment when exploration becomes more focused.

A stop and stand is commonly coupled with a challenge and is most effective when it comes as a great surprise to the patient, when it is unheralded, when it confronts severe mentalizing with an alternative perspective, and when the maneuver 'trips' the patient's mental processes and halts them in mid-flight.

The therapist calls a halt and seeks to stimulate reflection about an aspect of the session that has become muddling, perplexing or appears to indicate that the patient is making massive assumptions and basing decisions on them. Challenge should always be accompanied by the exploration of the patient's underlying feeling state; it is not a cognitive analysis of the logic of the dialogue. It is the point at which the therapist can go no further without questioning the patient's perspective that is being used to explain his experience and justify his stance but which in the end may induce action rather than discussion.

The complaining patient
A patient complained throughout the session that no one understood his problems. He had made a number of written complaints about the ill-treatment that he had received from mental health professionals whom he felt had never believed his reports of neglect

---

Box 9.8 Stop and stand

- Persist and decline to be deflected from exploration
- Steady resolve
- Convert deceit into frank truth
- Identify affect attached to action
- Ensure 'here and now' aspects are included in the challenge

as a child and so had not taken his problems seriously. Because he could function to some extent and was gainfully employed they had told him that he was all right and didn't need further help. As he talked about this he continually pointed out to the therapist that she didn't understand, and treatment with her was going to be useless.

Therapist: So I suppose that if I don't understand it will make it difficult for you to come to see me, especially if it means to you that I am not going to take your problems seriously (a basic mentalizing intervention linking the theme to the therapist/patient relationship and the consequential anxiety)?

Patient: (challenging tone): You can't understand because you have never experienced what I have. You weren't ill-treated as a child were you? I think I will have to go to one of those user groups where everyone has had the same experience. At least they might know how I feel.

Therapist: How do you know? (A challenging tone)

Patient: How do I know what?

Therapist: That I never experienced emotional neglect as a child?

Patient: Well you didn't.

Therapist: But what makes you say that?

Silence

Therapist: You feel very strongly that all these mental health professionals should not have made assumptions about you being OK and not needing help. But when it comes to you making assumptions about me and basing your attitude to me on those assumptions it is somehow OK. I am someone who can be dismissed as just another person who will not be able to understand because you assume that I have not experienced neglect.

Patient: That's different.

Therapist: In what way is it different?

Patient: It is.

Therapist: Is it? How come you make a formal complaint to the hospital board because other people have made assumptions about your difficulties and then acted on them? You seem to be doing the same thing to me.

The reader may feel that the therapist was becoming a little too challenging in this session but the therapist felt strongly that this was a core element of the patient's difficulties to the extent that as soon as he found his underlying feelings problematic he became dismissive of others without reflection, lost the ability to mentalize moment-arily and as result left therapeutic relationships with his feelings unaddressed and holding a grudge that no one understood him. The session continued to focus on this area. The stop and stand had reinstated some reflection on the part of the patient whose mostly pre-conscious assumption about the therapist was now conscious and 'on-the table' for discussion as something that might stimulate feelings that would lead him inexorably towards leaving therapy and repeating his previous interactions with therapists, and possibly writing a further letter of complaint. The therapist moved on to identify the fears the patient had of never being understood and his current feeling that the therapist would never be able to understand his wish to be understood as a person who had his own needs and desires, who required support and emotional care, and who needed help.

Stop and stand is only effective over the long term when used prudently. Excessive stop and stand disrupts the flow of a session and challenge employed too frequently is counterproductive. Therapists must use their judgment about when a gross assumption has been made or pseudomentalizing is gaining hold and is likely to result in a serious distortion of the process of therapy or in further acting out by the patient. Challenges should not be made in an unpleasant manner or with anger, but they require the therapist to persist and to decline from being deflected from exploration—'bear with me, I think we need to continue trying to understand what is going on'. The therapist maintains a steady resolve to examine the problem—'I can understand that you want me to move off this discussion about what you are doing but I do not think that would be right because . . .'.

Stop and stand may be necessary to reduce threats to therapy integrity, for example, when anti-social aspects of a patient's function predominate and justification of dangerous or illegal actions mount one on top of the other or the therapist becomes unclear about the veracity of a patient's story.

The well-dressed patient

A 26 year old male patient on probation for fraud attended the session looking distinctly different in appearance. Instead of his usual slightly 'unkempt look' he was wearing designer jeans and fashionable shoes.

Patient: How do you like my new look?

Therapist: You do look very different, I must say. What has happened to change things?

Patient: I just decided to buy some new stuff and to make myself look good. My grandmother gave me some money (said hurriedly).

Therapist: That was kind of her. And you decided to spend it on clothes. You do look good, but can you think about what made you begin to think about yourself a bit differently and want to present yourself to me and to others looking clean and well-dressed?.

Patient: I think that most of you just see me as a bad person and I am more than that.

The session continued in this way but gradually the therapist became pre-occupied with two thoughts. First, she felt that the patient might have stolen the clothes and that his explanation of money from his grandmother was specious; and second, that he had done it to present himself nicely to her. Eventually she brought her preoccupations in to the session as sensitively as she could.

Therapist: Going back to when you said that most people only see you as being bad, I wonder if one problem for you is that because people know you have been to prison for fraud you fear that everything you do makes them think that you might have committed further fraud. A bit like me thinking that you might have got your new clothes in that way rather than from your grandmother.

Patient: Do you?

Therapist: It did occur to me that something like that might have happened, particularly if you wanted to look good to come here.

Patient: So you don't really trust me then, do you? You think I stole them, don't you?

Therapist: I don't know how you got them, but you have said very little about your grandmother since you started in therapy, so she has 'come out of the blue' for me. Why don't you tell me more about her and what led her to give you some money?

Patient: You won't believe me anyway.

Therapist: I think that we have to face the fact that you have committed fraud using credit cards and been to prison for it and so if you suddenly appear with expensive things then people are going to be suspicious. That is something that you are going to have to live with for a time at least. But first let's consider what you expected me to think, especially since you have never mentioned your grandmother before. To me she is a fictional person.

In this vignette the therapist is trying to balance honesty about her state of mind with reflection about how this affects her responses in therapy. She has been candid and expressed her own assumptions whilst stopping and standing to allow the patient to begin further exploration of what is in his mind and what he understands might be engendered in the mind of the other. In fact in this case the patient's grandmother had visited from the north of England and given him some money which he had spent on his appearance. The key area for further examination turned out not to be the patient's dishonesty but his attachment to the therapist and his wish to present attractively to her.

There are times when a patient is blatantly dishonest or attempts to gloss over obvious deceit and at those times therapy itself is under threat. Initially it is important to convert frank deceit into a clearly stated truth. Until this has been done it is impossible to continue therapy.

Deceit is interesting from the perspective of mentalization. To deceive effectively an individual must have a capacity to understand the mind of the other person and to be able to predict what he will and will not believe and under what circumstances. To this extent the anti-social patient may have a highly tuned capacity of mentalizing, but it is our experience that this apparent ability is actually highly restricted and rarely generalizable to complex interpersonal situations. Anti-social patients are able to mentalize some specific mind states; for example, the exploitative patient easily picks up the subjective state of the dependent borderline patient and tunes in to her needs. Able to understand her underlying feelings he exploits her for his own ends, initially stimulating an erroneous trust and a misguided affection. An unequal relationship follows which deteriorates at the point at which the borderline patient expresses more complex mental states and feelings which the anti-social patient fails to understand and cannot react to other than with violence or coercive action to bring his partner back to a position in the relationship which he does understand. These relationships are dangerous for the dependent borderline patient and interfere with treatment if the relationship is between two patients who have met through group therapy. More sinister for treatment is the psychopathic patient who has the ability both to charm and to 'read minds' effectively but misuses this in serious exploitative or even sadistic behaviour. In common with other treatments we have no answer to this problem although we have discussed some of the underlying mind states leading to violence elsewhere (Fonagy, 2004).

Boundary violation

An intimate relationship between two or more patients creates severe difficulties for therapists and other patients, and there is no single correct response that meets all situations but this is a 'stop and stand' situation. The open reporting of such events has to be encouraged if they are to be explored within treatment, otherwise, if they occur, they are likely to be conducted in secret, which distorts the dynamics of group therapy even further. A hidden couple within a group acts like a foreign body, unknown and quiescent but dangerously infective if left for too long without exposure and detoxification. An identified couple allows the group to react and to consider their responses and to address the effect that it has on them and the group. Thus our first response to a relationship between two participants is to ask them to discuss openly the development of their relationship and its effect on their involvement in treatment and their understanding of its effect on others. From a mentalizing perspective the problem is that the formation of a pair rigidifies mentalizing across a whole group and may precipitate chronic pseudomentalizing—'I think that it is nice that they have met each other so why do we need to worry about it'; or even teleological thinking—'Good for them—at least they have got something really good from the group that they can take home!'. Under these circumstances the therapist has to recruit other members of the group and force the group to move from a 'dialogue of the deaf' to a mentalizing discussion.

Once all avenues have been explored and it becomes clear that the relationship is to continue, a stop and stand associated with an impasse should take place (see Box 9.9).

The boundaries of treatment are reiterated along with an understanding of the patients' position towards it—'You feel that your relationship has helped

> ## Box 9.9 **Stop and stand—dealing with an impasse**
>
> - Clarify your boundary (should be a repetition of boundary agreed when therapy began) whilst giving your understanding of patient's position in relation to it—'I think that you continue to attend simply so that you can force me to watch you deteriorate but I can't continue to do that. We need to tackle this'.
> - When all avenues explored state impasse—'As far as I can tell we are going round in circles. When I say something you simply dismiss it as rubbish and whilst I am willing to accept that it sometime is, I cannot accept that it always is'.
> - Recruit group members to recognize impasses and shift from 'dialogue of the deaf' to a mentalizing discussion.
> - State own position—'If we can't get around this I may have to say that treatment has failed and should finish'.
> - Monitor countertransference to ensure no acting out by therapist.

you, and I understand that it has made you feel happier. Our concern is that the special relationship that you have together will not only interfere with your ongoing treatment but also distort the treatment of the other patients in the group who are excluded from your special relationship. I realize that your view is that it may have little effect on what you decide to do but our experience is that things can go wrong for everybody and so we will have to consider discharging you both from treatment with the proviso that you may return to treatment if the relationship ends or you both want to reapply for treatment after 6 months when we could consider you for different groups'.

Basic mentalizing

There are a number of basic mentalizing techniques, which we have grouped together as 'stop, listen, look' and 'stop, rewind, explore'. These *aide de memoire* 'catchphrases' refer to the actions of the therapist as he tries to reinstate a mentalizing process in the session. The minds of both patient and therapist need to stop and/or re-wind to understand better the process that has been going on. Equally, the techniques can be applied to the content of the dialogue and the therapist may ask a patient to 'stop, rewind, and explore' his narrative as well, particularly if he glosses over detail and avoids describing underlying affects. The purpose of both strategies is to reinstate mentalizing when it has been lost or to promote its continuation in the furtherance of the overall goal of therapy which is, to reiterate, to encourage the formation of a robust and flexible mentalizing capacity that is not prone to sudden collapse in the face of emotional stress. As a session moves forward it is sometimes necessary either to pause to consider and to explore the moment or to move it back to retrace the process or re-examine the content.

Stop, listen, look

As an individual or group session unfolds the therapist needs to listen constantly for non-mentalizing processes and interactions. Indicators of poor mentalizing, such as failure to respond to feelings expressed by others, dismissive attitudes, trite explanations, or lack of continuity of dialogue, suggest that the therapist needs to stop, listen, and look. To do so he holds the group or individual session in a suspended state whilst investigating the detail of what is happening by high-lighting who feels what about whom, and what each member of the group

---

Box 9.10 Stop, listen, look

During a typical non-mentalizing interaction in a group or individual session

- ◆ Stop and investigate
- ◆ Let the interaction slowly unfold—control it
- ◆ Highlight who feels what
- ◆ Identify how each aspect is understood from multiple perspectives
- ◆ Challenge reactive 'fillers'
- ◆ Identify how messages feel and are understood, what reactions occur

---

Box 9.11 Stop, listen, look—questions

- ◆ What do you think it feels like for X?
- ◆ Can you explain why he did that?
- ◆ Can you think of other ways you might be able to help her really understand what you feel like?
- ◆ How do you explain her distress/overdose?
- ◆ If someone else was in that position what would you tell them to do?
- ◆ Recruit—Gemma is obviously angry. Can anyone help her with this, because I wonder if beneath it she is beginning to feel ignored.

understands about what is happening from his own perspective. On the one hand, the ther-apist has to be active about this exploration of the current state of the group or individual session (see list of common questions p 132), but, on the other hand, he must also listen to the responses carefully to piece together the complexity of the interactions and to make sense of the affective process that is interfering with each person's capacity to think about himself in relation to the others. Once the group has worked around the 'stop' point it can move on. It is only when mentalizing is seriously disrupted that a 'stop, rewind, explore' takes place.

Stop, rewind, explore

The difference here is that the therapist has to stop the group or individual session and to insist the session rewinds to a point at which constructive inter-action was taking place. The therapist has to take control of the group, rewind, and with the steady resolve of stop and stand, to explore, whilst moving forward frame by frame. To do so he has to retrace the steps of the group and halt at a point when patients were able to think about themselves and others con-structively, albeit with some difficulty.

Stop, rewind, explore should be implemented as soon as the therapist thinks the group or individual session has become uncontrolled and/or is in danger of rapid self-destruction; for example, patients walking out or enga-ging in inappropriately aggressive discourse.

The suicidal patient

A patient talked in a group about how suicidal she felt and about her plans to take an overdose. The group, with the help of the therapist, worked hard with her to under-stand what had precipitated her negative and destructive state of mind, in which she felt no one cared if she lived or died, and that she had anyone or anything to live for. Many attempts to help from other members of the group were rebuffed and it was apparent that the frustration of the group was building up. Before the therapist could control this and highlight the underlying frustration the following interaction took place:

Box 9.12 **Stop, rewind, explore**

- Let's go back and see what happened just then.
- At first you seemed to understand what was going on but then . . .
- Let's try to trace exactly how that came about.
- Hang on, before we move off, let's just rewind and see if we can under-stand something in all this.

Patient to the suicidal patient: I am fed up with all this. Whatever we say it is no good. Why don't you put everyone out of your misery and just do it?

Immediate silence in the group.

Therapist: That is a serious thing to say (stop), and I suspect that whilst you mean it at this moment it has come out of somewhere which we will all regret and so we had better go back (rewind) to see how we have reached this point in which one of us doesn't care if someone else lives or dies (explore).

Patient: So it will all be my fault I suppose now when she takes an overdose.

Therapist: No (stand). We are going to go back to see what has happened that has led you to be so frustrated that you don't care if she takes one or not (stop). Actually I don't think that it is like you and so perhaps we can start with going back to the point at which you began to feel frustrated (rewind). When did you first feel like that (explore)?

When implementing a 'stop' the therapist may initially use exploratory probes in an attempt to help the patient reflect. We have called these opening statements 'labelling with qualification', and they commonly bridge the gap between basic mentalizing and interpretive mentalizing.

Labelling with qualification ('I wonder if . . .' statements)

Labelling with qualification or 'wondering' statements can sound woolly and be received as irritatingly uncertain ('how should I know, you are supposed to be the therapist') but when used appropriately can propel a session forwards to further discussion and revelation. The mentalizing stance of 'not-knowing' implies that the therapist will 'wonder' more often than he 'knows', but it is important that if he 'knows' he does not 'wonder'. In our experience a therapist who 'wonders' too much is in danger of not letting a patient share his perspective and creating a false interaction—the patient understands the therapist's underlying subjective state of mind even if it is not openly expressed and reacts to it unconsciously, constructing a 'pretend' interaction in which both patient and therapist are tentative whilst both are certain.

'I wonder if . . .' statements are important to ensure that the patient discovers what he is feeling (he should not be told what he is feeling—see p 93). The manifest feeling may be labelled without qualification but the therapist's task is to identify the consequential experience related to that feeling. This is where labelling with qualification is important. Examples of therapist comments used to label with qualification are given in Box 9.13.

Transference tracers

Transference tracers are immediate links from the content and process of the session either to the patient/therapist relationship, an inward movement, or to the patient's life outside, an outward movement, but they do not have the depth and complexity of mentalizing the transference. They are a significant and necessary aspect of interpretive mentalizing and point the way towards mentalizing the transference. The aim of tracers is to move therapy towards the here-and-now aspect of interpersonal interactions. They are always current, do not link the past to the present, or move therapy from the present to the past, but link the present outside to the current in treatment, or conversely move the current emotion in the session to the outside life of the patient. Depending on the intensity of emotion within a session, transference tracers moving inwards from the outside may link to the treatment facility ('. . . like you feel about the department'), the treatment itself ('. . . just as you feel about the programme'), the therapy ('. . . I guess that mentalizing can become an equal pain'), the session ('. . . just as it is today') and sometimes the therapist himself ('maybe you feel the same about me').

As a general principle we assume that linking statements using the trajectory of departmental building at one end to therapist himself at the other represent an increase in interpersonal emotional intensity. The therapist has to choose the

---

Box 9.13 Labelling with qualification ('I wonder if . . .' statements)

- Explore manifest feeling but identify consequential experience— 'Although you are obviously dismissive of them I wonder if that leaves you feeling a bit left out?'
- 'I wonder if there are some resentments that make it hard for you to allow yourself to listen to rules. Let's think about why the rules are there?'
- 'I wonder if you are not sure if it's OK to show your feelings to other people?'

Box 9.14 Transference tracers—always current

- Linking statements and generalization—'That seems to be the same as before and it may be that . . .'; 'So often when something like this happens you begin to feel desperate and that they don't like you'
- Identifying patterns—'It seems that whenever you feel hurt you hit out or shout at people and that gets you into trouble. Maybe we need to consider what happens in you at those times.'
- Making transference hints—'I can see that it might happen here if you feel that something I say is hurtful'.
- Indicating relevance to therapy—'That might interfere with us working together'

intensity of the link he makes at any given moment. This will depend on how much he wants to heighten the tension and the emotion of the session. The 'hotter' the session the more advisable it is to link to the lowest level of intensity for a few moments to test whether the patient can easily tolerate greater intensity before moving towards the higher levels. Once direct links have been made to the therapist you are in the realm of interpretive mentalizing.

A summary of typical aspects of transference tracers is provided in box 9.14.

The involved patient

A patient talked extensively about her relationships with other women and bemoaned the fact that they always ended in acrimony after a few months. She felt that a pattern repeated itself with her becoming more and more dependent until she felt trapped and compelled to escape, which usually occurred by her blaming her partner for problems.

Patient: I told her that she didn't care about me. She said that she did but she doesn't. If she did she would have come after me. She never did though and nor did any of the others even though I was upset and angry.

Therapist: I was thinking that maybe you will feel very involved in treatment and it will make you feel trapped or that we aren't bothered about you. Then you will want to get out. I'll have to remember that we should come after you and contact you if that occurs if we are to help you come back.

Patient: Don't think it will happen here.

Therapist: Hope not but at least we know what to do if it does.

Patient: Hmmm.

The intolerant patient

Patient: I don't like it if I don't know what people are thinking. I avoid them or ignore them by going quiet and keeping my own thoughts to myself. I don't share if someone else doesn't. It's dangerous.

Therapist: So if you don't know what I am thinking it might interfere with therapy if you just go quiet and keep things to yourself?

Patient: I get angry and I won't talk about anything if I don't know what the other person is thinking.

Therapist: Tell me a bit more about that. What happens to make you feel you don't know what the other person is thinking? Has there been a time today when you have felt like that?

Interpretive mentalizing

Any interpretation should be used with caution. The basic structure of an interpretive intervention involves presenting an alternative perspective on what the patient has said. Normally it follows extensive elaboration of the experience which the patient described. Elaboration, as we have already described, involves the enriching of a description in collaboration with the patient. Thus when the patient described feeling angry about something the elaborative work identifies connected emotions, perhaps of anxiety or shame, and might link to a more complex and detailed depiction of the experience. For example, an initial statement about feeling in a rage with a manager becomes elaborated as having felt deeply anxious about being criticized and a clear depiction of the perceived facial expression and bodily posture of this man which was seen as threatening and undermining. While it is not the aim of elaboration to mentalize the patient's reaction, in interpretive mentalizing the therapist is asked to link the patient's reaction to a state of mind in a causal sequence. In the scenario just described a simple interpretation might be to link the patient's rage reaction to the fear of criticism with a simple statement such as 'Well, perhaps you felt frightened that you were going to be criticized and that made you just walk out in a rage'. The aim is to elaborate the interpretation together with the patient to try and recruit the patient to take a joint look at how they were acting in the situation, using mental state language to make sense of their actions for both themselves and the therapist.

The steps in interpretive mentalizing are: (1) clarification and elaboration of both emotion and experience; (2) identifying the failure of mentalization and encouraging active mentalization around the same theme; and (3) presenting an alternative view or perspective. For example, the patient reports on a painful argument with the partner where she was beaten up following an intense attack of possessiveness and jealousy on her part that ended in accusations of duplicity on the part of the partner. In clarifying the experience the therapist is able to elicit from the patient how her inability to understand the partner's behaviour had totally persuaded her that he had cheated on her. The therapist recognizes this as psychic equivalence and an indication of failure of mentalizing the partner. While it is possible that the partner was unfaithful, this is by no means the only possibility. In elaborating the patient's mental state, it becomes clear how the partner's lateness triggered a terror of abandonment that in turn led to a sense of overwhelming jealousy and possessiveness. It also becomes clear that the likely impact of this on the partner is not at all evident to the patient.

> The therapist gently says 'I've no way of knowing how John felt, but it sounds to me as though you just didn't know how to stop 'going on at him' as you put it.
>
> **Patient:** 'No, I just couldn't stop. There was nothing that he could say that would reassure me.

Therapist: I wonder how someone might feel when nothing they could say could deal with the situation?

Patient: I guess they would feel helpless, like I did.

Therapist: Is that all that they would feel?

Patient: No, I guess they would also feel very frustrated and angry.

Therapist: Do you think John felt frustrated and angry?

Patient: He must have done; that's why he hit me.

Therapist: But I don't think that you were aware of that at the time. I don't think you knew what effect you were having on him.

Patient: No, I just felt I had to go on and on, I had to get some reassurance, otherwise I was going to go mad.

Therapist: It sounds to me as though you felt very desperate indeed, is that right?

Patient: Yes, I was totally desperate, I thought I was going to lose him and I'd be alone again.

Therapist: It's my guess that when you feel so desperate you stop being able to think about the effect you are having on the other person. You just have to make sure that they are there and somehow when you go on at them it makes you feel that they are there, and that's reassuring.

Patient: It's like punching something to make you feel real, or cutting yourself or hitting your head on the wall.

Therapist: So maybe you 'wouldn't leave off', as you said, to make sure that you weren't left alone, and perhaps in that way even being hit was in a funny way reassuring for you.

Patient: Yes, it makes you feel real.

Dynamic therapists will inevitably raise a question concerning psychological defences such as displacement, projection, projective identification, disavowal and so on. Within MBT we consider defences to be part of normal mental activity and do not give it a special or specific place in our technique or our training. Defences are ways of thinking that in some way or another distort reality in the service of reducing unpleasure, or at least this is Freud's classical formulation. Within MBT, mentalizing defences is simply identifying the way a person may be avoiding or exaggerating a particular experience in order to make life easier for themselves in some way. A simple example follows to illustrate.

The patient, obviously upset, comes into his session and says to the therapist 'What's the matter with you today then?'

Therapist: What is it about me that makes you wonder if something is the matter?

Patient: Well you just look miserable.

Therapist: I wasn't aware that I was particularly, but again, what was it about me that made you think I might be?

Patient: I don't know. Everyone looks miserable to me today.

Therapist: Well you know, I had the same thought that you look rather miserable today. You look as though you have been crying.

Patient: I don't really want to talk about that.

The aim here is not for the patient to recognize that they were being defensive or understand the reason for their defensiveness; the therapist uses her understanding of the way defences work to help the patient back on the road to a fuller experience of their subjectivity. The same approach applies to other defences.

Mentalizing the transference

We are often asked by both psychoanalytic and non-psychoanalytic colleagues if MBT recommends using the transference. Our standard reply is 'it all depends what you mean by that phrase'. If you mean, do we focus on the therapist–patient relationship in the hope that discussion concerning this relationship will contribute to the patient's well-being, the answer is a most emphatic yes. If by using the transference you mean linking the current pattern of behaviour in the treatment setting to patterns of relationships in childhood and current relationships outside the therapeutic setting, then the answer is an almost equally emphatic no. Whilst we might well point to similarities in patterns of relationships in the therapy and in childhood or currently outside of the therapy, the aim of this is not to provide the patient with an explanation (insight) that they might be able to use to control their behaviour pattern, but far more simply as just one other puzzling phenomenon that requires thought and contemplation, part of our general inquisitive stance aimed to facilitate the recovery of mentalization.

Thus when we talk about mentalizing the transference, this is a shorthand term for encouraging patients to think about the relationship they are in at the current moment. It aims to focus the patient's attention on another mind, the mind of a therapist, and to assist the patient in the task of contrasting their own perception of themselves with how they are perceived by another, by the therapist or indeed by members of a therapy group. The emphasis is on using the transference to show patients how the same pieces of behaviour may be experienced differently and thought about differently by different minds. For example, the patient's experience of the therapist as persecutory and demanding, destructive and cruelly critical is one perception amongst many others.

It may be a valid perception given the patient's perception of the therapist's behaviour, but there are alternative ways of seeing how the therapist behaves. Once again the aim is not to give insight to the patient as to why they are distorting their perception of the therapist in a specific way but rather to engender curiosity as to why, given the ambiguity of interpersonal situations, they choose and stick to a specific version. In wondering why they might be doing this, we hope to help them recover the capacity to mentalize and in so doing give up the rigid, schematic psychic equivalent teleological way of interpreting their subjectivity and others' behaviour. Thus whilst we look at the motivation that the person might have for manifesting a particular type of 'transference', the reason behind such exploration is as always the encouragement of a thinking stance.

Perhaps the best way of explaining how MBT uses transference is to outline the six steps of an MBT transference interpretation (see Box 9.15). The first step is the validation of the transference feeling. The danger of the classical approach to the transference is that it might implicitly invalidate the patient's experience. The individual who feels the therapist to be persecutory and is functioning in a psychic equivalent mode is not helped by their experience 'being interpreted away' as part of a distortion, as, for example, it might be implied by the therapist's assertion that the patient insists on imposing a victim/victimizer type of dyadic relationship on his therapeutic experience.

Box 9.15 **Steps in MBT transference interpretations**

- ◆ Validation of transference feeling
  - Feeling is not crazy, it is real and legitimate
- ◆ Exploration of transference
  - Use techniques of exploration and elaboration above
- ◆ Accept enactment (if any)
  - Being drawn into transference is normal, admit it, draw attention to it
- ◆ Collaboration in arriving at interpretation
  - Use inquisitive stance to engage patient in inquiry
- ◆ Alternative perspective from therapist
- ◆ Follow patient reaction with next interpretation
- ◆ Journey more important than the destination

Thus the first step of a transference interpretation is ensuring that the patient feels that their feeling is real and legitimate, in the sense that there must be good reasons, normally to be found in the actions of the therapist, why they experience the therapist in a specific way.

> **Patient:** You don't care about me. For you I'm just work and even as work I'm boring and uninteresting.
>
> **Therapist:** I'm not sure what I have done but I must have done something, perhaps in the last few minutes or before, that makes you so convinced of that. Do you have any idea what I might have done?
>
> **Patient:** I saw you stifling a yawn and before then you looked at your watch.
>
> **Therapist:** You may be right. I wasn't aware of stifling a yawn but I do recall looking at my watch. Perhaps the way you are feeling at the moment it is inconceivable that there could be another explanation for me looking at my watch other than finding you a burden.

The second step is exploration of the transference. The transference, like any other interpersonal experience, in psychotherapy with a borderline patient needs thorough exploration. The techniques of elaboration and exploration that we have discussed above apply to transference feelings too. The therapist is ill-advised to accept at face value the initial report of an experience, however intense. It is important to explore the complexity of the transference feelings reported. For example, if the patient reports feeling angry or frustrated, what other feelings accompany these? Is it disappointment in the therapist or a sense of humiliation at being stuck with someone who appears unable to help, or perhaps even pleasure at having shown up the therapist to be inadequate? Similarly the facts from the patient's perspective must be clarified. The events which generated the transference feelings must be identified. The behaviours that the thoughts or feelings are tied to need to be made explicit, sometimes in painful detail. The therapist should remember not to mentalize the behaviours at this point, i.e. explain them or link them to subjective experience. This can inadvertently have the effect of invalidating the patient's experience. It is more important to trace actions to feelings in the sense of exploring the emotional impact of what the therapist or the patient did rather than the putative reasons behind them. In this context the most important goal may be to identify how the absence of mentalizing or indeed the absence of the possibility of mentalizing may be part of the patient's transference experience.

The third step is accepting enactment. Most of the patient's experiences in the transference are likely to be based on reality, even if on a very partial connection to it. Mostly this means that the therapist had been drawn into the transference, and acted in some way consistent with the patient's perception of her. It may be easy to attribute this to the patient's 'manipulativeness' but this would be completely unhelpful. On the contrary, the therapist should explicitly acknowledge even partial enactments of the transference as inexplicable voluntary actions that she or he accepts agency for. Drawing attention to such actions may be particularly significant in modelling to the patient that one can accept agency for involuntary acts and that such acts do not invalidate the general attitude which the therapist tries to convey. This may be essential in overcoming the patient's teleological stance where only actions are felt to be meaningful.

In the above sequence the therapist admitted to looking at her watch but not to stifling a yawn. Perhaps a more effective way of dealing with the situation would have been for the therapist to respond in the following way:

> I am not aware of having yawned but I can quite easily imagine that I might have done without noticing. I can see why that would upset you. It would probably upset me as well in the same circumstances. I am sorry for upsetting you but I wonder if the conclusion you drew that I was bored is the only possible one. What do you think?

Step four is collaboration in arriving at an interpretation. Transference interpretations must be arrived at in the same spirit of collaboration as any other form of interpretive mentalizing. The metaphor we use in training is that the therapist must imagine sitting side-by-side with the patient, not opposite. They sit side-by-side looking at the patient's thoughts and feelings, where possible both adopting the inquisitive stance. Thus the patient's anger and frustration, and the feelings of humiliation that surround it, become a target of joint inquiry.

> You were so quick to assume that I was bored with you when you thought that I yawned. I wonder why you were so quick to assume that I could lose interest in you so quickly. It seems surprising to me given how well we have been working together recently.

The therapist hopes that the patient will engage in this process but of course often the patient may just repeat what they already asserted. This reaction, however, can in turn become a subject of inquiry.

> **Patient:** Of course you were bored. It's obvious.
>
> **Therapist:** I am puzzled not only by how obvious it is to you but also by how hard it is for us to look at alternative explanations. Why do you think it is that it is so hard to think of any other possibility, even if what you think is true?

The fifth step is for the therapist to present an alternative perspective. Mostly the therapist leads the patient to consider an alternative perspective on their transference reaction. The key aim is the mentalization of the patient's transference experience. In the specific example that we are considering it is really not important to find out why the patient reacted with such anger. It is the failure of mentalization which the anger signals that must be the focus of the therapist's work.

> **Therapist:** What I might feel if someone looked at their watch whilst I was talking to them is that they wanted to be somewhere else. Was that part of what you were feeling?
>
> **Patient:** I am so boring. I always feel that you don't want to be with me and that you would rather be somewhere else.
>
> **Therapist:** I see. So when you saw me look at my watch you might have thought that I would rather be doing something else than be here with you?
>
> **Patient:** I thought I had lost you. I felt that you had gone, that you had abandoned me.
>
> **Therapist:** Now I understand why you got so angry. As we have seen before, it is very hard for you when those abandonment feelings start. You feel you have to do something.
>
> **Patient:** Sometimes I just hit out and this time I just hit out at you, but mostly it just works out that I hit out at myself. I end up being the one who suffers.
>
> **Therapist:** I guess that when you get angry with people they might sometimes withdraw even further.
>
> **Patient:** I'm sure they do but I can't help it. That feeling that I have been left is just too strong. I'm terrified that one day you will just leave me.

The sixth step is monitoring the patient's reaction and trying to interpret the patient's reaction to the interpretation. As insight is not the aim of the intervention, the transference interpretation by the therapist is not the end of the process. In fact a simple assertion by the therapist about how one may understand the patient's reaction will close down mentalizing rather than facilitating its further activation. The therapist thus explores the patient's reaction to the intervention as the final step of mentalizing the transference. In the present example the therapist may say:

> It strikes me that perhaps you feel relieved by being able to talk about these strong feelings that accompany your conviction that one day I will leave you.

At this stage the therapist is in step one of the process of mentalizing the transference again and has to start by validating the patient's conviction that the therapist will one day totally abandon him, showing that they recognize it is not a crazy but a real and legitimate feeling that has its own roots in other thoughts and feelings that the patient has, which have not yet been made explicit and need to be mentalized.

We hope that we have illustrated here that in our approach to transference interpretation it is not the particular type of content that needs to be elicited; it is the engaging in the process of uncovering the way the mind works that is relevant. It is going on a journey of discovery with the patient that we believe to be the helpful part of the intervention, and it is going on a journey rather than arriving at any specific destination that the patient and therapist should have as their shared goal.

Chapter 10

Mentalizing and group therapy

Group psychotherapy is a powerful context to focus on mental states of self and others. It stimulates highly complex emotional interactions which can be harnessed for all patients to explore the subjective understanding of others' motives whilst reflecting on their own motives. Inevitably this feature of the programme is one of the most difficult aspects of treatment for borderline patients who have the task of monitoring and responding to 6–8 minds rather than being able to focus on only two as in individual therapy. Herein lies the danger of group psychotherapy. The level of complexity and the sophistication of mentalizing required for group interaction means that conditions are optimal for things to fly out of control as attachment systems become over-stimulated and rigid schematic representations of others are rapidly mobilized. As such, group psychotherapy may become highly iatrogenic stimulating mental withdrawal, a collapse in mentalizing and action rather than verbalization—the very antithesis of its aim. First and foremost the therapist has to ensure that iatrogenic effects are minimized.

There are two main types of groups in our programme—explicit mentalizing groups using explicit mentalizing exercises, and implicit mentalizing groups using implicit mentalizing process. To understand the focus and aims of these two types of groups it is important to understand the difference between explicit and implicit mentalizing even though the two are intrinsically linked and neither can exist without the other. To complicate matters further, explicit mentalizing techniques may occasionally be used in implicit mentalizing groups and explicit mentalizing groups are, in part, inevitably using implicit mentalizing. Over the trajectory of treatment explicit mentalizing activity becomes more implicit whilst implicit mentalizing process, at first somewhat reduced, becomes less hesitant, less distorted, and increasingly automatic.

Explicit mentalizing

We mentalize explicitly most of the time. We are continuously thinking and talking together about our emotional states and thoughts and about those of others, particularly our partners and close friends and colleagues. As clinicians we talk about our patients' beliefs, desires, wishes, feelings, and motives on a daily basis and, for the most part, ask our patients to join us in doing so. When we talk to others we tend to focus on the here and now (identifying what someone experiences at the moment) but we also mentalize ourselves and others within different time frames. We ask ourselves and others if we have experienced anything similar before ('I know this feeling and it is familiar to me') and think about our mental states at the time ('why did I feel this then?'). We anticipate future mental states too, wondering how we will feel if we do something or how someone else will feel if we say something. Hopefully we move seamlessly between these different time zones as we use hindsight to find foresight and to facilitate more effective ways of managing similar situations over time.

In keeping with our moves around time frames we can mentalize within a narrower frame and the scope of our reflection is reduced to the immediate moment or to include only recent mind states and events. Alternatively we can hark back to distant past history and wonder about our upbringing, our parental relationships and use this to explain our current experience. We develop a narrative—a story about our mental states—and in the end the widest context for understanding any mental state is a full autobiography.

Explicit mentalizing group

The explicit mentalizing group is run on a weekly basis, lasts for one and half hours, follows a programme over 10–14 weeks and continues as a slow open large group. We have only organized this within the day hospital programme and it is not part of the research based intensive out-patient programme. Nevertheless it may be useful as an introduction to mentalizing and as a pre-treatment phase to mentalization based treatment. This has yet to be assessed. Those readers who are well-versed in psychoeducation techniques will have no difficulty with the basic aspects of an explicit mentalizing group, but it is essential that the dialogue is not 'educational' in the sense of telling the patient what he needs to know or how to deal with problems but is instructive in so far as it stimulates the patient to consider the overall process of mentalizing, its relationship to his difficulties and its contribution to his success or failure in managing emotional interactions, which are the primary aims of the group.

There are a number of principles guiding our explicit mentalizing groups (see Box 10.1).

Introductory session

Method
The group leader begins with an introduction to the concept of mentalizing covering a number of areas (see Box 10.2).

Box 10.1 Explicit mentalizing group

- ◆ Exercises are arranged in sequence progressing from emotionally 'distant' to more personalized.
- ◆ Introduce exercises using personal experience when group cohesive
- ◆ Develop exercises to ensure that there is a focus on:
  - Self or other
  - Perceptions and experiences of others about self
  - Perceptions of self about others.
- ◆ Exercises may run over a few weeks

Box 10.2 Psychoeducation for explicit mentalizing group

- ◆ Definition in simple everyday terms
- ◆ Discuss implicit and explicit mentalizing
- ◆ Difference between mentalizing and intellectualization, rationalization and other cognitive processes
- ◆ Influence of emotional states on mentalizing
- ◆ Illustrate introduction with examples from personal experience to normalize reduced capacity, for example, loss of temper in meeting
- ◆ Give examples from everyday intimate relationships, for example, marital rows

Discussion

Participants are asked to consider times when they think someone else has lost the capacity to mentalize (note that this is often easier for patients than being asked to describe a situation in which they have lost the ability). Then ask them how the person regained his capacity. Ensure that you ask the group to comment on each others' stories. Only personalize the discussion if you feel that the group has become cohesive and it is safe to make it more intimate.

Alternatives

Ask someone who has been in the group for a number of sessions to define mentalizing and to expand on his definition.

Understanding personal characteristics

Method
Provide photographs from newspapers and magazines of people on their own. Ask the group to pick a picture and to suggest the personal characteristics that they think the person might have. Remind the group that characteristics can be positive and negative and that people tend to have a mix of both.

Discussion
Ask each person in turn why he has chosen the characteristic and ask him to give the reasons to the rest of the group. Identify whether the group agrees that the characteristic sounds likely, e.g. a sports star being competitive; a model being self-obsessed. If not, why not?

Stimulate discussion about how such a characteristic might develop and what advantages and disadvantages it might have for the individual and others, for example, a sports star with a strong competitive streak might do well in competitions, but if this is maintained in all social situations it might alienate people.

Alternatives
If the group is working well together ask a few participants to describe one of their own characteristics. Get others to agree or disagree with their self assessment ensuring that they outline their reasons and give examples from the treatment process; for example, I don't think she is very patient because in the group last week . . .

Understanding attitudes

Method
Ask the group to suggest an attitude someone holds towards them. You may need to help them by giving examples, e.g. argumentative, submissive, dependent, dismissive, controlling.

Discussion
How do those attitudes help and hinder their relationship? What can change the attitude? Why did the attitude develop? Has the attitude affected them positively or adversely and how do they manage the situation?

Alternatives
Describe one of their own attitudes. Ask them to outline how the attitude developed and what effect it has on them now. How does it affect others' reactions to them? Do others in the group recognize this attitude?

Specify their attitude to police, social workers, psychiatrists, therapists and other professionals or officials. Expand their views and ask what might help them change their attitude. Do they see the person as an individual or identify them as someone who takes on the characteristics attached to their official role?

Describe attitudes to family members with discussion as above.

Understanding motives

Method
Ask the group to consider an episode in their life in which family or friends are talking together and then something happens which they find hard to explain. For example, a patient described talking to her sister and mother when her younger brother walked out of the room having been silent throughout the conversation.

Discussion
The group need to ask for information related to the story which might help them decide on possible underlying motivations for the action. In this example information about the topic of conversation, the relationships within the family, and the usual interaction between the patient and her brother might help towards understanding his motivation.

Alternatives
Consider using an episode from the treatment programme. Unexplained actions are common, particularly in implicit mentalizing groups, and so exploration of an incident may be done within the explicit mentalizing group away from the 'heat of the kitchen'.

Participants give an example of an interaction in which they have felt hurt or wounded by someone they liked or trusted. The example can be from the treatment programme. The discussion centres around their reaction and their understanding of why the hurtful person acted as he did. What were his reasons? Why is he like that? What are the possible explanations? How did the patient react and would a different reaction been better?

This scenario can be reversed with the patient talking about an incident in which they have been hurtful to someone else. Again, the example can be from the treatment programme.

Understanding emotions

Method
Ask each member of the group to describe the prevailing mood of someone they know well and with whom they have a relationship; for example, close friend, mother, father, partner. Try to help them recognize that moods are complex by asking them to describe in detail what they mean by anger, happiness, sadness, etc.

Discussion

How do they explain the individual's prevailing mood? Does it affect their relationship? Is the primary contribution to their mood from current or past experience? Have they noticed anything that can change the mood? Can the patient help the person change their mood?

Alternatives

Ask the participants to identify their own prevailing mood. Suggest they verify it with other members of the group. Divergence should be explored. Discussion as above.

What makes me 'me'?

Method

Most people tend to think of themselves as having some unique characteristics. Ask participants to give one or two aspects of themselves which they think differentiates them from others in the group. Do not ask them initially to comment on unique features of others in the group.

Discussion

Each member spends a few minutes describing what makes me 'me' and contrasts it with other members of the group. Then ask participants to suggest common factors between themselves and others in the group. If this seems too difficult ask for contrasts and similarities with family members. Ask other members to comment and whether they agree or disagree and if so why. How have my unique features developed over time and what have been the most significant contributing factors?

Alternatives

This group can be difficult for participants and you can consider asking them to write down what makes me 'me' instead of having to talk about it straightaway. Participants can then read out what they have written.

Understanding self through other

Method

Ask group members to pick someone else in the group and to describe how they think that person actually sees them. Consider basic aspects of how people see each other as well as more complex psychological elements, for example, smart, sense of humour, capable, caring. Ask other members to comment on whether they think the description is accurate or not and if not why not. Ask the person whose mind is being described not to comment on the accuracy or to react to the description until the group has explored the portrayal. Instead, ask him to write down what is being said for later comment.

Discussion

Once the group have worked on the description ask the person to give his actual understanding of the person and to balance what has been said with his actual opinion. Discuss how difference in understanding might have developed. Is this because things are not spoken about and remain hidden and, if so, why are they not talked about? Is there something important about how he sees the other patient that has been missed?

Alternatives

Ask participants to describe how they think someone who loves them or hates them sees them. How would that person describe them if he was in the group now? How has he come to that opinion? Has the patient contributed to development of the viewpoint?

Implicit mentalizing

We mentalize implicitly within all our interactions, and yet when we try to grasp the essence of the process it slips away into explicit mentalizing which at once destroys the quintessence of the implicit process. Implicit mentalizing is automatic, procedural, natural and below the level of consciousness. We are not aware that we are doing it and yet, when asked, we know that we are constantly monitoring ourselves and others intuitively, without thought. We base our opinions of others on our subjective experience of them as much as on our rational deductions—'He seems very nice but there is something about him I don't trust'. There is a balance that we naturally draw as implicit and explicit mentalizing intertwine together, more like the 'double helix' than a continuum in its complexity, forming a multifaceted psychological understanding of ourselves, coding our relationships, representing them and re-presenting them as we interact.

When we mentalize others we monitor their mental states, taking in their point of view, their emotional states and a sense of their underlying motives. We intuitively reflect and, when things go smoothly, our mind states change in tune with theirs and we take pleasure in the interaction as it progresses and we see that not only have we changed them a little but we too have been changed. We respond to their presentation of themselves and to their re-presentation of us. Yet if we tried to do all this explicitly all of the time we would stumble and become like an automaton, emotionless and non-human. Nobody would like us or feel warm towards us, experiencing us as hollow and without depth, and we would be unable to feel close to them. Communication of our inner self would have been interrupted.

When we mentalize ourselves implicitly we are in more treacherous territory being in a position to remain unchallenged and subject to distortions via our defences or even dominated by our explicit rationalizations. Yet we are aware that there is something about us that we know is us—a sense of self rooted in our emotional states. This is the 'I' that can represent 'me'. To reflect on our emotional states we have to remain in them and to do so we have to maintain an experience of our sense of self, otherwise our emotions will overwhelm us. We need to identify the inner experience, modulate it, understand its narrative—where has it come from, what is its meaning—and express it. Not surprisingly it is a tall order for treatment to target this process and this may have led some, perhaps wisely, to dismantle implicit mentalizing into smaller elements and to target them rather than the overall process in treatment. Hence there are a number of conceptual cousins, for example empathy, self-awareness, introspection, reflectiveness, mindfulness, all of which overlap but, at risk of over-generalizing, tend to be present centred whereas implicit mentalizing is at once present- past- and future-centred.

Implicit mentalizing group

The broad aims of the implicit mentalizing group are in keeping with our definition of implicit mentalizing discussed above, that is, to promote mentalizing about oneself, mentalizing of others and mentalizing of relationships.

Inevitably promoting implicit mentalizing takes time and we suggest that a minimum time of 1 year is necessary to stimulate the process and to allow it to become embedded as a robust aspect of an individuals' psychological function within relationships. There are no short cuts.

Focussing on mentalizing in a slow open group requires the therapist to utilize many of the interventions already discussed in this chapter but there are some aspects that bear further discussion. First, the therapist, at times, has to take control of the group and he must be able to do this whilst remaining part of, the group. To this end he demonstrates that he is a participant in, and not an observer of, the group. Second, monitoring anxiety levels of both the whole group and the individuals in the group is necessary to ensure they are optimal and become neither too high nor too low—over-arousal results in the group or an individual becoming uncontrolled whilst inadequate expression of emotion and over-intellectual discussion prevent development of mentalizing in the context of 'hot' attachment interactions. Both situations are to be avoided and it is to this end that the therapist maintains control of the group. Third, interventions that aim to increase mentalizing within the group in the immediacy of the moment form the key to constructive development of the group. But whilst we stress most of the work takes place within current mental reality this does not mean there should be no consideration of past and future which may themselves be part of current reality as a patient explores his own meaning and considers himself in future situations. Full mentalizing transfers hindsight to foresight, allowing us to predict our future responses and those of others; current sight allows us to understand the past within a new frame allowing what was implicit to become explicit. So the therapist needs to keep an eye on each patient's history as it is played out in the group and on the trajectory of the group itself as it develops its own history.

Monitoring anxiety and control of the group

Control of group work is implemented through the use of stop and stand and the therapist's insistence on focusing the group on what is happening in the moment. The addition of a 'rewind' and slow movement forward exploring what has happened ensure that the group remains focused and does not become a free associative group but one that remains purposefully centred around mentalizing. As a general principle the therapist must intervene and take control of a group at the point at which either the group engages in non-mentalizing, for example pseudo mentalizing, indicating anxiety levels may be falling too low, or when mentalizing collapses completely with, for example bizarre mentalizing or sudden rigid representations of others, suggesting anxiety levels are too high. The same principles apply to any loss of his own capacities so when his own ability to understand what is going on in himself and in the group diminishes he should at least stop, listen, look at himself if not the group. Typical examples in a group indicating a decrease in mentalizing are listed in Box 10.3. Such changes may occur within an individual, between one or more individuals, or across the whole group itself.

The patient who walks out

A common and sometimes unpredicted indicator of a failure of mentalizing due to high anxiety is a patient walking out—action instead of words. When this

Box 10.3 **Indicators of breakdown of mentalizing in groups**

- Overt or covert hostility
- Active evasion
- Non-verbal reactions—sullen, walking out, restlessness
- Gross assumptions about the therapist or another patient
- Taking words literally

occurs the therapist needs to take charge and not leave the situation hanging. Until proven otherwise patients walk out because they need to get their mind back and can only do so when alone and out of reach of others' minds. Once they have retrieved their mind they can come back in to the group and we have found that patients who leave a group return, more often than not, after a few minutes. Nevertheless the therapist may have to leave the group briefly to help the patient return or suggest that another group member goes to the patient's aid.

> Patient D was silent in the group right from the start of the session. Questions were rebuffed with 'don't know' until everyone stopped asking how she was. Suddenly the patient got up and walked out saying 'This is crap'.
>
> **Therapist:** Try to stay if you can (no effect; the patient continued towards the door and left).
>
> **Patient A:** Oh dear.
>
> **Patient B:** At least that means we don't have to keep thinking about what is wrong with her.
>
> **Patient C:** I was beginning to feel fed up with her sulking around in the corner anyway.
>
> **Patient E:** Me too.
>
> **Therapist:** Her silence was difficult for us all (active participant). I think someone might go to see if she can come back though. Can anyone go?
>
> No volunteers from the group and a steadfast silence.
>
> **Therapist:** I'll go and be back in just a moment.
>   The therapist gets up and leaves the room and returns within a minute (a structural intervention with teleological meaning both to the remaining patients and to Patient D).
>
> **Therapist:** I have just seen her and suggested that she come back in as soon as she can. Hopefully she will be able to shortly. Maybe we had better go back because it seems that everyone felt there was something wrong right from the beginning of the group and yet we didn't know how to help. Who can start us off, maybe by letting us know what they feel is wrong with Patient D at the moment?
>   Here the therapist takes clear charge of the group and then focuses on what has happened by first taking the group back to the beginning to explore what has actually been going on within people's minds but has been unspoken.
>
> **Patient C:** I don't really care. She doesn't want to tell anyone so why should we bother.
>
> **Therapist:** It is difficult to care if someone doesn't seem to try and it is easy to give up.
>
> **Patient C:** She gave up, not us. She walked out. We've got other things to talk about and she has left so she has lost her chance.

Therapist: I think we gave up just before Patient D walked out. But the problem we now face is that she probably feels we don't care and have given up on her and if we leave it perhaps we are confirming that for her (basic mentalizing in the moment).

Patient B: I think that she walked out to upset us.

The therapist then insisted that the group discuss this aspect by asking about why Patient D would want to upset the group. During this dialogue Patient D returned to the group and so the therapist first summarized what had been said during the patient's absence to continue the focus on the group's initial understanding of why the patient had walked out, namely to upset everyone. This was soon found to be erroneous.

Specific interventions to promote mentalizing

We have already discussed basic mentalizing interventions and these are used in the groups. Here we give a few pointers for the therapist about ways in which he can stimulate implicit understanding of one's own and others' motives.

Explore understanding of each other

Therapists familiar with common group techniques and systemic questioning will have little difficulty in recognizing the interventions described here. The aim of each intervention is to stimulate a mentalizing process and to generate different perspectives on the fly as each patient is confronted with a number of different understandings of himself and pressured to reconsider his own view of himself, his effect on others and others' effect on him. To promote this the therapist may do a number of things. He may:

- Focus on what a patient is saying asking him to clarify and expand (this should not become an analysis of the individual within the group)—'Can you tell us a bit more about that?' 'Has something like this happened before?'

- At the moment of uncertainty expand the dialogue by asking other patients about their understanding of what is being said—'What is your under-standing of what Patient A has been saying?' 'How do you understand her suicidal feelings?' 'Can anyone else help with this?'

- Generalize the problem and find commonality between patients—'Has anyone else experienced this?' or if necessary direct a question to a patient who you know has similar problems—'Patient A, I think you know about this sort of problem'.

- Return to a topic sensitively or if necessary stop and stand whenever the group dismisses something that is manifestly important, for example, an overdose or self-harm by a patient—'I think that we must try to spend a bit more time on what has been going on that led Patient D to take an overdose. Patient D, can you tell us a bit more about things following the last group when we talked a bit about how difficult things were for you'.

◆ Generate a group culture of enquiry about motivations questioning different aspects of the same events and diverse understanding of the same dialogue—'Perhaps none of us has the complete answer to this and we are all experiencing a different component'—whilst ensuring that all viewpoints have equal validity until an integrated perspective is developed.

◆ Insist that patients consider others' perspective and work to understand some one else's point of view—'How can you explain her view to yourself?' 'Why does he feel as he does about this?'

◆ Challenge inappropriate certainty and rigid representation—'You seem to think that only you have the right view here and how you see Patient C is the only aspect of her that has any credence. That seems very dismissive of others' views.'

◆ Express directly his own feeling about something that he believes is interfering with group progress. For example if the therapist feels frustrated about the lack of help the group is giving to a patient he might say how frustrated he is—'I feel very frustrated by this and I am not sure what to do about it but everyone seems fed up today and unable to contribute. Can someone help me with what is going on?'

All these interventions require the active therapist stance described in Chapter 7. It is anticipated that the therapist feels comfortable working within a group and is able to withstand being dismissed, ridiculed or made to feel useless. If there are two therapists in the group their interactive relationship is significant. Crucially the therapists should be able to disagree respectfully and question each other in front of the patients. A united front is less important than demonstrating attempts to understand each others' perspective.

Joint therapists

Therapist A made an intervention in a group which led to complete silence. Therapist B found that her mind went blank as her colleague was intervening and so she wondered if this had happened to the patients' minds too. But she did not pass over the responsibility to the patients to tackle what had happened but took on the active therapist role.

Therapist B: As you were talking I became a bit unclear about what you were saying. Can you say it again or perhaps say it in a different way?

(The alternative intervention of asking the rest of the group what has happened to their minds is likely to make them feel that they should be responding in a way that at this moment they cannot. We ask therapists to consider their role in creating problems within the group before placing the problem out to the whole group)

Therapist A: Oh. It wasn't very clear and that might be because I wasn't clear in my own mind. I was suggesting that the group seem to have difficulty with listening to each other and I seem to have made it a little worse!

Therapist B: Well I was certainly having difficulty listening to what you were saying. Do you have any suggestion about what is behind that problem?

(Therapist B now tries to get Therapist A to expand what he is saying. Hopefully he will be able to do so.)

Therapist A: I was thinking that it might be related to the argument that went on yesterday between Patient C and Patient F that has not been mentioned but seemed to me to be very important. I have thought a lot about it since yesterday and still can't understand what happened to lead to the argument.

At this point Therapist A has focused the group and has been helped to do so by Therapist B. It is now wise to move from inter-therapist activity to the whole group.

Therapist B: What do other people think about this? Perhaps that argument has made people a bit uncertain and wary even.

Patient C: I still feel cross about it all and now Patient F is not here anyway. Obviously she doesn't want to face up to what she did.

Silence

Therapist A: Does anyone know what Patient C is referring to about what Patient F can't face?

This last intervention is a typical example of how the therapist attempts to get the group to express what they have in mind about what Patient C has in mind. In fact it turned out that they all had something different in mind about what Patient F could not face, which left them a little more sympathetic to her plight after it was discussed simply because they concluded that she was worried that everyone would 'gang up' on her.

In conclusion, the technique of clarifying and exploring between patients should become the baseline of the group process and interpretive mentalizing occurs only when this process is well established. In this group Therapist A went on to suggest:

Therapist A: I am beginning to think that we might have been a bit relieved that Patient F didn't come so that we didn't have to revisit what happened but then felt a bit guilty believing it was our fault she had stayed away and that might have led to the sense of wariness.

At this point one of the patients 'confessed' that she had phoned Patient F to say that she thought it might be better if she didn't come to the group to let things cool off.

Chapter 11

Frequently asked questions

We are grateful to all those who have asked questions during our training sessions, at conferences, in clinical discussions, in e-mails and even by carefully crafted snail mail. We provide a selection here of the most frequently asked questions. In the spirit of mentalization these have caused us to modify our training, re-think aspects of our treatment programme and add to our theoretical base. Unashamedly, we have taken from others what we think might enhance the understanding and treatment of BPD, and we hope that others will feel free to take what they think is useful from us. The motivations behind questions are often complex, personal, even political, and commonly aim further than simple fact finding, and so we include some of the more mischievous questions because often they have provoked lively discussion and stimulating debate. Inevitably we are often unable to answer questions satisfactorily which we hope will act as a stimulus to others to take the subject further rather than act as a stick with which to beat us.

Is this a new therapy?

This question may be phrased in many ways, often focusing on areas of commonality between the practice of MBT and other therapies—'Isn't that the same as . . .?' People mention all sorts of therapies, some of which we know little about, but it is clear that therapists often recognize aspects of their own treatment whether they are cognitively, dialectically, dynamically or humanistically trained. So . . .

No, it is not a new therapy and many of the techniques are a reiteration of well-known basic therapy practices such as support, empathy, exploration and challenge. To this extent we are a generic therapy with a focus on techniques that address the core difficulties of BPD. MBT is a focus for therapy rather than a specific therapy in itself.

MBT is a dynamic therapy using the relationship and the process of therapy as a key mechanism of change. The major difference between MBT and other dynamic therapies is that we suggest modulating some common therapy techniques such as genetic transference interpretation and enhancing others such as focusing on the current state of mind of the patient and giving more explicit support.

Isn't mentalization the same as cognitive therapy?

No. That is not to say that cognition is not a key part of MBT but cognition is a key part of any psychosocial treatment, even behavioural therapy. In fact we cannot imagine a psychological therapy that is able to bypass the patient's cognition. If we consider mentalization deficit to be merely a deficit of cognition and MBT as a remedial intervention close to skills training then the similarity between CBT and MBT will be more than superficial. The difference between the approaches is in the model of the mind or perhaps the model of human behaviour which MBT and CBT draw. CBT with its roots in social learning theory has a model of behaviour which specifically eschews dynamic determinants. Cognitions can be changed directly, it is assumed, without the need to focus on underlying determinants other than reinforcement contingencies. MBT, perhaps because of the psychoanalytic roots of the approach, has a model of mind that is at heart dynamic. MBT therapists are encouraged to think dynamically about the patient's experience. This includes assumptions about unconscious thoughts, feelings, wishes and desires and the patient's struggle with these complex experiences in the context of the interpersonal pressures of their lives, particularly attachment relationships. We are well aware that many CBT approaches are quite dynamic in the mental model they propose. Equally, MBT explicitly discourages therapists from focusing on unconscious determinants in their interventions (although not in their thinking about the patients). Thus it is perhaps disingenuous to try and create too sharp a distinction between these approaches as practised, but there are substantial practical differences.

MBT uses some CBT strategies simply because they are in themselves encouraging of mentalizing, especially at the beginning of treatment when psycho-education and motivational interviewing are important. There is no specific use of problem-solving skills which often include teaching fundamental communication skills; there is no attempt to delineate cognitive distortions outside the current patient–therapist relationship or to focus on behaviour itself; there is no explicit work on schema-identification; and finally there is no homework.

Isn't mentalization just supportive therapy?

Yes and no. It is supportive but not just supportive therapy. Additional active techniques are used (we recognize that supportive therapy also uses active techniques and is not simply a passive support of the patient but in fact a tech-nically difficult and somewhat under-rated treatment). We firmly believe that supportive work is necessary and that without it more active techniques are rendered less effective. In MBT support needs to be demonstrable within the teleological world of the patient within appropriate boundaries of therapy and not assumed to be taking place within the mental world because of the use of certain techniques.

Is mentalization really an analytic therapy?

MBT fits best into the plurality of analytic therapy with its emphasis on the patient–therapist relationship, understanding of dynamic processes and its move in treatment from conscious understanding to unconscious meaning. It differs in its greater emphasis on direct support, contractual structure, focus, modification of interpretive techniques and transparency of therapist.

Do you use validation?

Yes we do. But validation needs careful definition. It is an important theoret-ical and technical aspect of Dialectical Behaviour Therapy involving active observing, reflection and direct validation. The first two aspects of validation are common to every therapy and are an essential aspect of MBT. Direct val-idation requires the therapist to take a non-judgemental attitude, another essential aspect to all therapies, and search for the essential validity of the patient's experience and responses rather than its dysfunctional character-istics. It is direct validation that forms a crucial aspect of DBT. It is used to confirm the patient's experience and contingent response as being under-standable in a specific context. In MBT direct validation follows the same principles but the focus is on exploration rather than confirmation of the internal experience and on elaborating a multi-faceted representation based on current experience, particularly with the therapist. If a patient says 'I am a fool', the task of the therapist is to accept the statement and to promote explo-ration. The statement is a non-mentalizing self-judgement, and the therapist's task is to help the patient develop mentalizing, perhaps by suggesting that he, the therapist, might have done or said something to invoke the experience so that the raw statement becomes a more complex self-representation that can be worked on in the interpersonal domain. Reassuring the patient that he is not a fool will be ineffective and simply make him feel misunderstood, but saying something like, 'You have never appeared a fool to me but tell me what makes you say that at the moment' is both validating and offers an alternative perspective in order to promote mentalizing.

Is mentalizing the same as mindfulness?

No it is not. But they are overlapping constructs. Mindfulness is a construct originating in Zen Buddhist philosophy. It implies an acute orientation to current experience. Zen teaches that each moment is complete and perfect by itself and acceptance, toleration and validation, rather than change, should be the therapeutic focus. In its original sense it is not specific to mental states and as currently construed is equally applicable to the physical as to the mental world. However the central construct is the recognition that thoughts are just thoughts and that they are not 'you' or 'reality'. This recognition can free the patient from the distorted reality that thoughts can create. Thus mindfulness becomes a symbolic representation of mind and implies an attitude of openness and reflecting on whilst not reacting to, all of which are aspects of the mentalization construct. But mentalization is essentially relational and takes in experience of the other as well as experience of one's self and this helps distinguish these overlapping concepts. Further the time frame of mentalizing is broader in that mentalizing may invoke the past and the future as well as the present which is the focus of mindfulness. In general terms mindfulness cultivates mentalization.

Mentalizing does not seem specific to this therapy. All therapies promote mentalizing so what is so special about this?

Perfectly true. The only specific aspect of MBT is making the enhancement of mentalizing itself the focus of treatment. All therapies probably increase mentalizing indirectly, but in other therapies the therapist's aim is probably different, for example, to increase insight or to delineate schemas, and they are not aware that they are increasing mentalizing!

Mentalization theory blames the mother

Most certainly not! This question seems to arise because our developmental view gives some importance to the role of parents/carers and childhood experience in psychological development. Yet we consider a complex gene–environment interaction as the most likely cause of the reduction of mentalizing capacity in BPD. There is little doubt that both carers and children can disrupt the attachment relationship. This is not the same as apportioning blame to either of them and the influence of carers in psychological development is of particular importance in prevention strategies.

Does it matter if a patient has mixed therapies?

No! Cognitive interventions, dynamic therapy and expressive therapy can all be combined as long as the therapists meet to integrate their knowledge and understanding from a mentalizing perspective and mentalizing provides a coherent focus between all therapies. The danger is offering different therapies, targeting different symptoms or behavioural problems and failing to integrate the overall treatment. Many patients receive multiple treatments; for example, anxiety management, behaviour modification, expressive therapy and individual cognitive or dynamic therapy, but therapists have no contact with each other. We feel strongly that this type of treatment organization is inappropriate and the disaggregation of patient care in this way is antithetical to good treatment for BPD.

Do you use family therapy?

It depends on what you mean. We involve families, partners and carers in treatment plans as long as the patient agrees and we discuss with families and others how best to react to crises, what they can do to support treatment and how to reduce emotional interactions that escalate the problems for the borderline patient. We do not use formal family therapy itself as part of the treatment programme. In part this is because few of our patients live with their family. However we do ask family services to intervene using family work if a patient has children and child protection issues need to be considered.

Do I have to be an expert therapist already trained in a major model?

No! We have implemented MBT using generic mental health nurses. It is more important that practitioners are confident in basic communication with patients and experienced in appraising risk, e.g. suicide threats, potential violence, emergency admission, than being highly trained in complex therapy interventions. However, someone who is well trained in basic psychotherapy technique and familiar with mentalization needs to provide supervision.

What training do I need to implement MBT?

A very brief training is probably adequate if you are an experienced mental health professional to ensure that you modify your current technique to include a focus on mentalizing. A number of people have attended our 3-day training programme which covers theory and practice and uses videos to focus the discussion about technique. The use of video and audio recording of sessions followed by discussion with similarly trained colleagues is probably the best way forward to ensure adherence to the mentalizing focus.

What is the exact format of the out-patient treatment programme?

One individual session (50 minutes) plus one group session (90 minutes) per week with additional psychiatric care within the team; for example, for review of medication, reports, liaison with other professionals and crisis management. Therapists integrate treatment by sharing information in between sessions, by agreeing the primary active themes of the patient's problems and through regular joint supervision.

You use individual and group therapy. Is the individual therapy confidential?

The individual therapy session is confidential to the team and not solely to the individual therapist. The individual therapist meets with the group therapists and discusses the main themes of the sessions. The patient is aware of this. Thus the patient and individual therapist do not hold information secretly. The group therapists will not reveal information to the group about the patient which has arisen in the context of the individual session, but if the theme or information is important for treatment the patient will be encouraged by the individual therapist to talk about it in the group.

Do other personality disorders show reduced mentalizing?

Probably. But not in the same way as BPD. This remains an empirical question and needs further study. The commonest form of this question is whether MBT is useful in treatment of anti-social personality disorder (ASPD) perhaps because there remains no effective treatment for this group of individuals and practitioners struggle to manage such patients. The irony is that patients with ASPD show some enhanced, although compartmentalized, capacities in mentalizing but misuse their mentalizing. Treatment may therefore have to be focused not so much on increasing mentalizing capacity in this group but in removing the gratification from its misuse.

What is the evidence base for problems in mentalizing as a core feature of BPD?

There is an increasing evidence base for the significance of the attachment relationship in the development of a capacity to mentalize. There is also evidence that attachment relationships are disrupted in patients with BPD and that they have suffered significant environmental insults during development. We have reviewed this literature. In addition there is evidence that mentalizing is reduced in BPD but primarily when the attachment relationship is stimulated and when intersubjective interactions increase in complexity. However even under these circumstances mentalizing can be maintained in BPD by deactivating the attachment relationship. This might occur in behavioural terms by walking away from the situation so that you can think about something and someone else—leaving a therapy group for example and returning when you have 'got your mind back'. Nevertheless unequivocal evidence that individuals with specific attachment patterns in childhood develop BPD in adulthood remains unproven. The problem is that a direct link is unlikely and the complexity of the gene–environment interaction means that establishing specific links is far from easy.

Do you think your treatment works?

Yes and no. It is clear from all the data that we have collected and from our published randomized trial that some patients do well. A further out-patient randomized trial is nearing completion. Our drop-out rate is low. However, not all patients do well. At the point of writing we do not have clear predictors of response to treatment, which is a pity, but we do know that gender does not predict outcome and treatment is equally effective or ineffective, depending on the slant you want to take, in both males and females. Our studies are small and need independent replication. This is taking place and we can confirm that the drop-out remains low when MBT is applied elsewhere by other professional teams, but we do not yet have data on outcome.

Surely what you are doing is simply good practice?

Yes. We think that good practice in treatment of BPD requires a team using a coherent philosophy of treatment over the long rather than the short-term associated with a number of other non-specific features of organization such as structure, integration with other services available to the patient, clear communication, well-established crisis pathways and careful attention being paid to the attachment relationship. What needs to be established is what the effective ingredients of treatment actually are. We do not yet know if more specific aspects of therapy, in our case the focus on mentalizing, are the most important components.

Does the mentalizing therapist self-disclose?

Yes. But no more than you would in everyday interaction. We do not suggest that you talk to the patient about your life and personal circumstances. Indeed such disclosure serves little purpose. We do, however, recommend that tactful disclosure about what you are feeling is essential and an explanation of the reasons for your reaction is useful especially when challenged by the patient. Careful self-disclosure verifies a patient's accurate perception and underscores the reality that you are made to feel things by him which is an essential aspect of treatment. The patient has to know what he creates in you in order to understand himself. Complete failure to self-disclose is likely to lead to enactments on your part either by persistent interpretation or by inappropriate actions. Rigorous non-reactivity is iatrogenic, because it makes the patient panic as he tries to find himself in another mind and when he fails to do so there is collapse in his representational world just when he requires another mind to provide that representation which is so essential for his stability. It is for these reasons that we do not immediately reflect questions but answer them prior to exploring them.

Do you work with fantasy?

The use of fantasy and free association is not a major part of MBT, because the development of insight is not a primary aim of MBT. Working with fantasy is a technique used in insight orientated therapy as a way of understanding unconscious thinking. MBT is more concerned with pre-conscious and conscious aspects of mental function within the interpersonal domain. Fantasy itself is too distant from reality and we do not therefore encourage elaboration of the patient's fantasies about the therapist, because it is likely to be iatrogenic and to invoke pretend mode rather than increase elaborated representations linked to reality. We do, however, work with reality orientated fantasy, for example, exploring what the patient 'imagines would happen if . . .'. This enhances mentalization by forcing the patient to conjure representations of himself in different contexts and at a different time.

Do you ask patients to report dreams?

No, we do not ask patients to talk about their dreams. However, sometimes patients do. Needless to say, it is rarely productive to use free association techniques with this group of patients to elaborate the latent content of the dream images they report. There is an approach, however, which we have found helpful. If one considers the dream of a person who is struggling with mentalization in certain contexts not to be a disguised representation of unconscious thoughts and ideas but rather as an honest attempt to create self-reflective awareness, then these dreams can appear as meaningful communications. Thus a patient who dreams about being in an empty house or opening drawers and finding nothing in them or dreams of people with blank faces may be expressing an accurate perception of their mind as experientially empty of content. Similarly, repeated dreams about chaotic uncontrollable animals, wild horses, insects, serpents, birds, etc. depict an experience of mental content that refuses to be regulated. This hypothesis is worth mentioning, because often the therapist is able to relate better to the subjective experience of the dream if they have in mind the dream as a depiction of metacognition, that is, the patient's experiential relationship to the functioning of their own mind. In this context the emotional experience that is related often makes good sense. The patient reporting a dream where they find themselves in a crumbling building fearing its imminent collapse yet being unable to leave may be depicting for the therapist the sense in which they feel trapped in a mental world that they do not feel they can rely on and that could collapse at any time.

Further reading

On mentalizing and MBT

Allen, J. G. and Fonagy, P. (2006) *Handbook of Mentalization-Based Treatment.*
New York: Wiley.

Bateman, A. W. and Fonagy, P. (2004) *Psychotherapy for Borderline Personality Disorder: Mentalization Based Treatment.* Oxford: Oxford University Press.

Fonagy, P. and Bateman, A. W. (2006) Progress in the treatment of borderline personality disorder (editorial). *British Journal of Psychiatry, 188,* 1–3.

Fonagy, P. and Bateman, A. W. (2006) Mechanisms of change in mentalization-based treatment of BPD. *Journal of Clinical Psychology, 62*(4), 411–430.

On other therapeutic approaches to BPD

Gunderson, J. G. (2001) *Borderline Personality Disorder: A Clinical Guide.* Washington, DC: American Psychiatric Publishing.

Gunderson, J. G. and Hoffman, P. D. (eds) (2005) *Understanding and Treating Borderline Personality Disorder. A Guide for Professionals and Families.* Arlington: American Psychiatric Publishing.

Kernberg, O., Clarkin, J. F. and Yeomans, F. E. (2002) *A Primer of Transference Focused Psychotherapy for the Borderline Patient.* New York: Jason Aronson.

Krawitz, R. and Watson, C. (2003) *Borderline Personality Disorder. A Practical Guide to Treatment.* Oxford: Oxford University Press.

Lenzenweger, M. F. and Clarkin, J. F. (eds) (2005) *Major Theories of Personality Disorder* (2nd edn). New York: Guilford Press.

Linehan, M. M. (1993) *The Skills Training Manual for Treating Borderline Personality Disorder.* New York: Guilford Press.

Livesley, W. J. (2003) *Practical Management of Personality Disorder.* New York: Guilford Press.

Oldham, J., Skodol, A. E. and Bender, D. S. (eds) (2005) *Textbook of Personality Disorders.* Arlington: American Psychiatric Publishing.

Young, J. E., Klosko, J. S. and Weishaar, M. E. (2003) *Schema Therapy. A Practitioners Guide.* New York: Guilford Press.

Appendix

Checklist to be used in the clinical assessment of mentalization

	Note most compelling example	Strong evidence (+1)	Some evidence (+0.5)	Total score
In relation to other people's thoughts and feelings				
Opaqueness				
The absence of paranoia				
Contemplation and reflection				
Perspective-taking				
A genuine interest				
Openness to discovery				
Forgiveness				
Predictability				
Score				
Perception of own mental functioning				
Changeability				
Developmental perspective				
Realistic scepticism				
Acknowledgement of preconscious function				

Table (continued)

	Note most compelling example	Strong evidence (+1)	Some evidence (+0.5)	Total score
Conflict				
Self-inquisitive stance				
An interest in difference				
Awareness of the impact of affect				
Score				
Self-representation				
Advanced pedagogic and listening skills				
Autobiographical continuity				
Rich internal life				
Score				
General values and attitudes				
Tentativeness				
Moderation				
Score				

Categories of mentalizing capacity based on clinical assessment

Context	Score	Category
In relation to other people's thoughts and feelings		
	5.0–8.0	Very high (3)
	3.0–4.5	Good (2)
	1.0–2.5	Moderate (1)
	0.0–0.5	Poor (0)
Perception of own mental functioning		
	5.0–8.0	Very high (3)
	3.0–4.5	Good (2)
	1.0–2.5	Moderate (1)
	0.0–0.5	Poor (0)
Self-representation		
	3.0	Very high (3)
	1.5–2.5	Good (2)
	0.5–1.0	Moderate (1)
	0.0	Poor (0)
General values and attitudes		
	2.0	Very high (3)
	1.0–1.5	Good (2)
	0.5	Moderate (1)
	0.0	Poor (0)
OVERALL		
	9.5–12	Very high (3)
	6.0–9.0	Good (2)
	2.5–5.0	Moderate (1)
	0.0–2.0	Poor (0)

Self rating of MBT adherence

Use the outline here to monitor your implementation of mentalizing interventions. The initial domain of framework of treatment is primarily for use at the beginning of therapy, but you should check that you continue to keep to the framework reviewing your aims, crisis plan and formulation on a regular basis.

Framework of treatment

Yes	No	DK	My treatment is offered in a clearly structured context that is transparent to patients and treaters. (2)
Yes	No	DK	I have a clear hierarchy of therapeutic goals agreed with patient. (2)
Yes	No	DK	I have a crisis plan identified. (2)
Yes	No	DK	A case discussion has been organized where roles of other staff have been identified and the limits of confidentiality agreed. (1)
Yes	No	DK	My patient appears to understand the rationale of treatment and the purpose of group and individual therapy. (1)
Yes	No		I have explained the boundaries of therapy. (2)
Yes	No		I have arranged supervision either in peer group or with a senior practitioner. (1)
Yes	No		I have reviewed the patient's current relationships and social support network. (2)
Yes	No		I have reviewed medication or arranged for review with a colleague. The limits of medication prescribing have been defined. (1)
Yes	No		Assessment of mentalization has been completed. (1)
Yes	No		Diagnosis has been discussed with the patient. (1)
Yes	No		My formulation has been completed and been discussed with the patient and modified accordingly. (2)

Max = 18

Mentalization

Yes	No	I am taking a genuine stance of 'not-knowing' and attempting to 'find out'. (2)
Yes	No	I ask questions to promote exploration. (1)

Yes	No	In the session I ask about patients' understanding of motives of others. (1)
Yes	No	I use transference tracers in this session. (1)
Yes	No	I use transference interpretation to highlight alternative perspectives and not to give insight. (1)
Yes	No	I challenge unwarranted beliefs about me and patients' experience of self and other. (1)
Yes	No	I do not present the patient with complex mental states. (2)
Yes	No	I avoid simplified historical accounts of current problems. (2)
Yes	No	I avoid confrontation with patient when he is in psychic equivalence mode. (2)
Yes	No	I consider if the pretend mode of mentalization is present in the patient. (2)
Yes	No	I address reversibility of mental states. (1)

Max = 16

Working with current mental states

Yes	No	I attend to current emotions. (2)
Yes	No	I focus on appropriate expression of emotions. (1)
Yes	No	I link affect with immediate or recent interpersonal contexts. (1)
Yes	No	I relate understanding of current interpersonal context to appropriate recent past experiences. (1)

Max = 5

Bridging the gaps

Yes	No	My reflections aim to present the patient's internal state in a modified form. (2)
Yes	No	I give examples to the patient of his experience of psychic equivalence. (1)
Yes	No	I focus attention of patient on therapist experience without being persistently self-referent. (1)
Yes	No	I negotiate ruptures in alliance by clarifying patient and therapist roles in the rupture. (1)
Yes	No	I am trying to develop a transitional 'as if' playful way of linking internal and external reality in sessions. (1)
Yes	No	I judiciously use humour. (1)

Max = 7

Affect storms

Yes   No   I maintain a dialogue throughout the emotional outburst. (2)

Yes   No   When emotions are aroused I attempt to clarify the feeling and any underlying emotion without interpretation. (1)

Yes   No   I only begin to address possible underlying causes of the affect storm within patient's current life as the emotional state subsides. (2)

Yes   No   I identify triggers for the storm in patient's construal of their interpersonal experience immediately prior to it. (1)

Yes   No   I link affect storm to therapy process only after storm has receded. (2)

Max = 8

Use of transference

Yes   No   I build up over time to transference interpretation. (2)

Yes   No   I only use transference interpretation when therapeutic alliance is established. (1)

Yes   No   I do not use transference as simple repetition of the past. (1)

Yes   No   I use transference to demonstrate alternative perspectives between self and other. (1)

Yes   No   I avoid interpreting the therapeutic relationship as part of another relationship that the patient currently has or has had in the past. (1)

Yes   No   My transference interpretations are brief and to the point. (1)

Yes   No   I refrain from use of metaphor when the patient's mentalizing capacity is reduced. (2)

Yes   No   I do not focus on apparent conflict. (1)

Max = 10

How much overall adherence do I exhibit in this session?

Add up the number of YES answers multiplied by the weight of the item and divide by 64. You should get 80% overall. Add up the points for each section and divide by the maximum point for that section You should score at least 75% on all the domains.

Is my adherence across all domains?

Which area do I need to focus on in the next session?

References

Agrawal, H. R., Gunderson, J., Holmes, B. M. and Lyons-Ruth, K. (2004). Attachment studies with borderline patients: a review. *Harvard Review of Psychiatry, 12*(2), 94–104.

Allen, J. G. (2000). *Traumatic Attachments*. New York: Wiley.

Allen, J. G. (2006). Mentalizing in practice. In J. G. Allen and P. Fonagy (Eds.), *Handbook of Mentalization Based Treatments*. Chichester, UK: Wiley.

American Psychiatric Association. (2001). Practice guidelines for the treatment of patients with borderline personality disorder—introduction. *American Journal of Psychiatry,* **158**, 2.

Appelbaum, S. A. (1973). Psychological-mindedness: Word, concept and essence. *International Journal of Psycho-Analysis,* **54**, 35–46.

Arnsten, A. F. T. (1998). The biology of being frazzled. *Science,* **280**, 1711–1712.

Arntz, A. and Veen, G. (2001). Evaluations of others by borderline patients. *Journal of Nervous and Mental Disease,* **189**(8), 513–521.

Aveline, M. (2005). The person of the therapist. *Psychotherapy Research,* **15**, 155–164.

Baron-Cohen, S., Tager-Flusberg, H. and Cohen, D. J. (Eds.). (2000). *Understanding Other Minds: Perspectives from Developmental Cognitive Neuroscience*. Oxford: Oxford University Press.

Bartels, A. and Zeki, S. (2000). The neural basis of romantic love. *Neuroreport,* **11**(17), 3829–3834.

Bartels, A. and Zeki, S. (2004). The neural correlates of maternal and romantic love. *Neuroimage,* **21**(3), 1155–1166.

Bateman, A. W. and Fonagy, P. (1999). The effectiveness of partial hospitalization in the treatment of borderline personality disorder—a randomised controlled trial. *American Journal of Psychiatry,* **156**, 1563–1569.

Bateman, A. W. and Fonagy, P. (2001). Treatment of borderline personality disorder with psychoanalytically oriented partial hospitalization: an 18-month follow-up. *American Journal of Psychiatry,* **158**(1), 36–42.

Bateman, A. W. and Fonagy, P. (2004). *Psychotherapy for Borderline Personality Disorder: Mentalization Based Treatment*. Oxford: Oxford University Press.

Bateman, A. W. and Tyrer, P. (2004). Psychological treatment for personality disorders. *Advances in Psychiatric Treatment,* **10**, 378–388.

Beeghly, M. and Cicchetti, D. (1994). Child maltreatment, attachment, and the self system: Emergence of an internal state lexicon in toddlers at high social risk. *Development and Psychopathology,* **6**, 5–30.

Bohus, M., Haaf, B., Simms, T., Limberger, M. F., Schmahl, C., Unckel, C. *et al.* (2004). Effectiveness of inpatient dialectical behavioral therapy for borderline personality disorder: A controlled trial. *Behavioral Research Therapy,* **42**(5), 487–499.

Bowlby, J. (1969). *Attachment and Loss, Vol. 1: Attachment*. London: Hogarth Press and the Institute of Psycho-Analysis.

Bowlby, J. (1988). *A Secure Base: Clinical Applications of Attachment Theory*. London: Routledge.

Briere, J. and Runtz, M. (1988). Symptomatology associated with childhood sexual victimization in a non-clinical adult sample. *Child Abuse and Neglect*, 12, 51–59.

Chiesa, M., Fonagy, P., Holmes, J. and Drahorad, C. (2004). Residential versus community treatment of personality disorders: A comparative study of three treatment programs. *American Journal of Psychiatry*, 161(8), 1463–1470.

Clarkin, J. F., Hull, J. W. and Hurt, S. W. (1993). Factor structure of borderline personality disorder criteria. *Journal of Personality Disorder*, 7, 137–143.

Clarkin, J. F., Levy, K. N., Lenzenweger, M. F. and Kernberg, O. F. (2004a). *The Personality Disorders Institute/Borderline Personality Disorder Research Foundation randomized control trial for borderline personality disorder: Progress report*. Paper presented at the Annual Meeting of the Society for Psychotherapy Research, Rome, Italy.

Clarkin, J. F., Levy, K. N., Lenzenweger, M. F. and Kernberg, O. F. (2004b). The Personality Disorders Institute/Borderline Personality Disorder Research Foundation randomized control trial for borderline personality disorder: rationale, methods, and patient characteristics. *Journal of Personality Disorder*, 18(1), 52–72.

Cloitre, M., Scarvalone, P. and Difede, J. (1997). Post-traumatic stress disorder self- and interpersonal dysfunction among sexually retraumatized women. *Journal of Traumatic Stress*, 10, 437–452.

Damasio, A. R. (2003). *Looking for Spinoza: Joy, Sorrow, and the Feeling Brain*. New York: Harvest Books.

Dennett, D. (1987). *The Intentional Stance*. Cambridge, MA: MIT Press.

Department of Health. (2003). Personality disorder: No longer a diagnosis of exclusion. *Department of Health Publications*.

Farber, B. A. (1985). The genesis, development and implications of psychological-mindedness in psychotherapists. *Psychotherapy*, 22, 170–177.

Fonagy, P. (2004). Early life trauma and the psychogenesis and prevention of violence. *Annals of the New York Academy of Sciences*, 1036, 1–20.

Fonagy, P. and Bateman, A. (2006). Mechanisms of change in mentalisation based therapy with BPD. *Journal of Clinical Psychology*, 62(4), 411–430.

Fonagy, P. and Target, M. (2002). Early intervention and the development of self-regulation. *Psychoanalytic Inquiry*, 22(3), 307–335.

Fonagy, P., Steele, H. and Steele, M. (1991). Maternal representations of attachment during pregnancy predict the organization of infant–mother attachment at one year of age. *Child Development*, 62, 891–905.

Fonagy, P., Leigh, T., Kennedy, R., Mattoon, G., Steele, H., Target, M. *et al.* (1995). Attachment, borderline states and the representation of emotions and cognitions in self and other. In D. Cicchetti and S. S. Toth (Eds.), *Rochester Symposium on Developmental Psychopathology: Cognition and Emotion* (Vol. 6, pp. 371–414). Rochester, NY: University of Rochester Press.

Fonagy, P., Leigh, T., Steele, M., Steele, H., Kennedy, R., Mattoon, G. *et al.* (1996). The relation of attachment status, psychiatric classification, and response to psychotherapy. *Journal of Consulting and Clinical Psychology*, 64, 22–31.

Fonagy, P., Redfern, S. and Charman, T. (1997). The relationship between belief-desire reasoning and a projective measure of attachment security (SAT). *British Journal of Developmental Psychology*, 15, 51–61.

Fonagy, P., Target, M. and Gergely, G. (2000). Attachment and borderline personality disorder: A theory and some evidence. *Psychiatric Clinics of North America,* **23**, 103–122.

Fonagy, P., Gergely, G., Jurist, E. and Target, M. (2002). *Affect Regulation, Mentalization and the Development of the Self.* New York: Other Press.

Frith, U. and Frith, C. D. (2003). Development and neurophysiology of mentalizing. *Philosophical Transactions of the Royal Society of London B, Biological Sciences,* **358**, 459–473.

Gabbard, G. O. (2005). Mind, brain, and personality disorders. *American Journal of Psychiatry,* **162**(4), 648–655.

Gallagher, H. L. and Frith, C. D. (2003). Functional imaging of 'theory of mind'. *Trends in Cognitive Sciences,* **7**(2), 77–83.

Gallese, V., Keysers, C. and Rizzolatti, G. (2004). A unifying view of the basis of social cognition. *Trends in Cognitive Sciences,* **8**(9), 396–403.

Gergely, G. and Csibra, G. (2003). Teleological reasoning in infancy: The naïve theory of rational action. *Trends in Cognitive Sciences,* **7**, 287–292.

Gergely, G. and Watson, J. (1996). The social biofeedback model of parental affect-mirroring. *International Journal of Psycho-Analysis,* **77**, 1181–1212.

Gergely, G. and Watson, J. (1999). Early social-emotional development: Contingency perception and the social biofeedback model. In P. Rochat (Ed.), *Early Social Cognition: Understanding Others in the First Months of Life* (pp. 101–137). Hillsdale, NJ: Erlbaum.

Gidycz, C. A., Hanson, K. and Layman, M. J. (1995). A prospective analysis of the relation-ships among sexual assault experiences: an extension of previous findings. *Psychology of Women Quarterly,* **19**, 5–29.

Gilligan, J. (1997). *Violence: Our Deadliest Epidemic and its Causes.* New York: Grosset/Putnam.

Gunderson, J. G. (1996). The borderline patient's intolerance of aloneness: Insecure attachments and therapist availability. *American Journal of Psychiatry,* **153**(6), 752–758.

Gunderson, J. G. (2001). *Borderline Personality Disorder: A Clinical Guide.* Washington, DC: American Psychiatric Publishing.

Gunderson, J. G., Bender, D., Sanislow, C., Yen, S., Rettew, J. B., Dolan-Sewell, R. *et al.* (2003). Plausibility and possible determinants of sudden 'remissions' in borderline patients. *Psychiatry,* **66**(2), 111–119.

Gurvits, I. G., Koenigsberg, H. W. and Siever, L. J. (2000). Neurotransmitter dysfunction in patients with borderline personality disorder. *Psychiatric Clinics of North America,* **23**(1), 27–40, vi.

Hayes, S. C., Follette, V. M. and Linehan, M. (Eds.). (2004). *Mindfulness and Acceptance: Expanding the Cognitive Behavioral Tradition.* New York: Guilford.

Hopkins, J. (1992). Psychoanalysis, interpretation, and science. In J. Hopkins and A. Saville (Eds.), *Psychoanalysis, Mind and Art: Perspectives on Richard Wollheim* (pp. 3–34). Oxford: Blackwell.

Keller, M. B., Lavori, P. W., Mueller, T. I., Endicott, J., Coryell, W., Hirschfeld, R. M. *et al.* (1992). Time to recovery, chronicity, and levels of psychopathology in major depression. A 5-year prospective follow-up of 431 subjects. *Archives of General Psychiatry,* **49**, 809–816.

Kernberg, O. F. (1987). Borderline personality disorder: A psychodynamic approach. *Journal of Personality Disorders,* **1**, 344–346.

Kohut, H. (1971). *The Analysis of the Self*. New York: International Universities Press.

Koren-Karie, N., Oppenheim, D., Dolev, S., Sher, S. and Etzion-Carasso, A. (2002). Mother's insightfulness regarding their infants' internal experience: Relations with maternal sensitivity and infant attachment. *Developmental-Psychology, 38*, 534–542.

Lambert, M., Bergin A. E. and Garfield, S. (2004). Introduction and historical overview. In M. Lambert (Ed.), *Bergin and Garfield's Handbook of Psychotherapy and Behavior Change* (pp. 3–15). New York: Wiley.

Lieb, K., Zanarini, M. C., Schmahl, C., Linehan, M. M. and Bohus, M. (2004). Borderline personality disorder. *Lancet, 364*(9432), 453–461.

Linehan, M. (1986). Suicidal people: One population or two? *Annals of New York Academy of Science, 487*, 16–33.

Linehan, M., Comptois, K. A., Brown, M. Z., Reynolds, S. K., Welch, S. S., Sayrs, J. H. R. et al. (2002). *DBT versus nonbehavioral treatment by experts in the community: Clinical outcomes*. Paper presented at the Symposium presentation for the Association for the Advancement of Behavior Therapy, Reno, NV. Seattle: University of Washington.

Linehan, M. M. (1987). Dialectical behavioural therapy: A cognitive behavioural approach to parasuicide. *Journal of Personality Disorders, 1*, 328–333.

Linehan, M. M., Armstrong, H. E., Suarez, A., Allmon, D. and Heard, H. (1991). Cognitive-behavioural treatment of chronically parasuicidal borderline patients. *Archives of General Psychiatry, 48*, 1060–1064.

Livesley, W. J. (2003). *Practical Management of Personality Disorder*. New York: Guilford.

Lochman, J. and Dodge, K. (1994). Social cognitive processes of severely violent, moderately aggressive, and nonaggressive boys. *Journal of Consulting and Clinical Psychology, 62*, 366–374.

Lyons-Ruth, K. (1996). Attachment relationships among children with aggressive behavior problems: The role of disorganized early attachment patterns. *Journal of Consulting and Clinical Psychology, 64*, 64–73.

Marcel, A. (2003). The sense of agency: Awareness and ownership of action. In J. Roessler and N. Eilan (Eds.), *Agency and Self-Awareness* (pp. 48–93). New York: Oxford University Press.

McCallum, M. and Piper, W. E. (1996). Psychological mindedness. *Psychiatry, 59*(1), 48–64.

Meares, R. (2000). *Intimacy and Alienation: Memory, Trauma and Personal Being*. London: Routledge.

Meares, R. and Hobson, R. F. (1977). The persecutory therapist. *British Journal of Medical Psychology, 50*, 349–359.

Meins, E., Fernyhough, C., Wainwright, R., Das Gupta, M., Fradley, E. and Tuckey, M. (2002). Maternal mind-mindedness and attachment security as predictors of theory of mind understanding. *Child Development, 73*, 1715–1726.

Nelson, E. E., Leibenluft, E., McClure, E. B. and Pine, D. S. (2005). The social re-orientation of adolescence: a neuroscience perspective on the process and its relation to psychopathology. *Psychological Medicine, 35*, 163–174.

Nickell, A. D., Waudby, C. J. and Trull, T. J. (2002). Attachment, parental bonding and borderline personality disorder features in young adults. *Journal of Personality Disorder, 16*(2), 148–159.

Ogden, T. (1985). On potential space. *International Journal of Psycho-Analysis, 66*, 129–141.

Paris, J. (2000). Childhood precursors of borderline personality disorder. *Psychiatric Clinics of North America,* **23**(1), 77–88, vii.

Paris, J. (2004). Is hospitalization useful for suicidal patients with borderline personality disorder? *Journal of Personality Disorder,* **18**(3), 240–247.

Patrick, M., Hobson, R. P., Castle, D., Howard, R. and Maughan, B. (1994). Personality disorder and the mental representation of early social experience. *Developmental Psychopathology,* **6**, 375–388.

Phelps, E. A. and LeDoux, J. E. (2005). Contributions of the amygdala to emotion processing: From animal models to human behavior. *Neuron,* **48**(2), 175–187.

Preston, S. D. and de Waal, F. B. (2002). Empathy: Its ultimate and proximate bases. *Behavioral & Brain Sciences,* **25**(1), 1–20; discussion 20–71.

Russell, D. E. H. (1986). *The Secret Trauma: Incest in the Lives of Girls and Women.* New York: Basic Books.

Ryle, A. (2004). The contribution of cognitive analytic therapy to the treatment of borderline personality disorder. *Journal of Personality Disorder,* **18**(1), 3–35.

Sack, A., Sperling, M. B., Fagen, G. and Foelsch, P. (1996). Attachment style, history, and behavioral contrasts for a borderline and normal sample. *Journal of Personality Disorder,* **10**, 88–102.

Sanislow, C. A., Grilow, C. M. and McGlashan, T. H. (2000). Factor analysis of DSM-III-R borderline personality criteria in psychiatric inpatients. *American Journal of Psychiatry,* **157**, 1629–1633.

Sayar, K., Ebrinc, S. and Ak, I. (2001). Alexithymia in patients with antisocial personality disorder in a military hospital setting. *Israel Journal of Psychiatry Related Science,* **38**(2), 81–87.

Shea, M. T., Stout, R. L., Yen, S., Pagano, M. E., Skodol, A. E., Morey, L. C. *et al.* (2004). Associations in the course of personality disorders and Axis I disorders over time. *Journal of Abnormal Psychology,* **113**(4), 499–508.

Silk, K. R. (2000). Borderline personality disorder. Overview of biologic factors. *Psychiatric Clinics of North America,* **23**(1), 61–75.

Slade, A., Grienenberger, J., Bernbach, E., Levy, D. and Locker, A. (2005). Maternal reflective functioning, attachment, and the transmission gap: A preliminary study. *Attachment & Human Development,* **7**(3), 283–298.

Solomon, J. and George, C. (1999). *Attachment Disorganization.* New York: Guilford.

Spillius, E. B. (1992). Clinical experiences of projective identification. In R. Anderson (Ed.), *Clinical Lectures on Klein and Bion* (pp. 59–73). London: Routledge.

Sroufe, L. A. (2005). Attachment and development: A prospective, longitudinal study from birth to adulthood. *Attachment & Human Development,* **7**(4), 349–367.

Stanley, B., Gameroff, M. J., Michalsen, V. and Mann, J. J. (2001). Are suicide attempters who self-mutilate a unique population? *American Journal of Psychiatry,* **158**(3), 427–432.

Steimer-Krause, E., Krause, R. and Wagner, G. (1990). Interaction regulations used by schizophrenic and psychosomatic patients: Studies on facial behavior in dyadic interactions. *Psychiatry,* **53**(3), 209–228.

Stone, M. H. (1990). *The Fate of Borderline Patients: Successful Outcome and Psychiatric Practice.* New York: Guilford Press.

Teasdale, J. D., Segal, Z. V., Williams, J. M. G., Ridgeway, V. A., Soulsby, J. M. and Lau, M. A. (2000). Prevention of relapse/recurrence in major depression by Mindfulness-Based Cognitive Therapy. *Journal of Consulting and Clinical Psychology,* **68**, 615–623.

Trull, T. J. (2001). Structural relations between borderline personality disorder features and putative etiological correlates. *Journal of Abnormal Psychology,* **110**(3), 471–481.

Trull, T. J., Sher, K. J., Minks-Brown, C., Durbin, J. and Burr, R. (2000). Borderline personality disorder and substance use disorders: A review and integration. *Clinical Psychology Review,* **20**(2), 235–253.

Tyrer, P. and Bateman, A. (2004). Drug treatments for personality disorders. *Advances in Psychiatric Treatment,* **10**, 389–398.

Verheul, R., van den Bosch, L., Koeter, M., de Ridder, M., Stijnen, T. and van den Brink, W. (2003). Dialectical behaviour therapy for women with borderline personality disorder: 12-month, randomised clinical trial in The Netherlands. *British-Journal-of-Psychiatry,* **182**(2), 135–140.

Vermote, R., Vertommen, H., Corveleyn, J., Verhaest, Y., Franssen, M. and Peuskens, J. (2003). *The Kortenberg–Louvain Process-Outcome Study.* Paper presented at the IPA Congress, Toronto.

Watson, J. S. (2001). Contingency perception and misperception in infancy: Some potential implications for attachment. *Bulletin of the Menninger Clinic,* **65**, 296–320.

Wicker, B., Keysers, C., Plailly, J., Royet, J. P., Gallese, V. and Rizzolatti, G. (2003). Both of us disgusted in my insula: The common neural basis of seeing and feeling disgust. *Neuron,* **40**(3), 655–664.

Winnicott, D. W. (1956). Mirror role of mother and family in child development. In D. W. Winnicott (Ed.), *Playing and Reality* (pp. 111–118). London: Tavistock.

Winnicott, D. W. (1967). Mirror-role of the mother and family in child development. In P. Lomas (Ed.), *The Predicament of the Family: A Psycho-Analytical Symposium* (pp. 26–33). London: Hogarth Press.

Winnicott, D. W. (1971). *Playing and Reality.* London: Tavistock.

Wollheim, R. (1995). *The Mind and its Depths.* Cambridge, MA: Harvard University Press.

Zanarini, M. C., Frankenburg, F. R., Hennen, J. *et al.* (2005). Psychosocial functioning of borderline patients and Axis II comparison subjects followed prospectively for six years. *Journal of Personality Disorder,* **19**, 19–29.

Zanarini, M. C., Frankenburg, F. R., Hennen, J., Reich, D. B. and Silk, K. R. (2004). Axis I comorbidity in patients with borderline personality disorder: 6-year follow-up and prediction of time to remission. *American Journal of Psychiatry,* **161**(11), 2108–2114.

Zanarini, M. C., Frankenburg, F. R., Hennen, J. and Silk, K. R. (2003). The longitudinal course of borderline psychopathology: 6-year prospective follow-up of the phenomenology of borderline personality disorder. *American Journal of Psychiatry,* **160**(2), 274–283.

Zanarini, M. C., Williams, A. A., Lewis, R. E., Reich, D. B., Vera, S. C., Marino, M. F. *et al.* (1997). Reported pathological childhood experiences associated with the development of borderline personality disorder. *American Journal of Psychiatry,* **154**, 1101–1106.

Zlotnick, C., Mattia, J. and Zimmerman, M. (2001). Clinical features of survivors of sexual abuse with major depression. *Child Abuse and Neglect,* **25**(3), 357–367.

Index